Speech Retarded and Deaf Children: their psychological development

45824

WITHDRAWN

23 APR 2025

COLLEGE LIBRARY

**Please return this book by the date stamped below
- if recalled, the loan is reduced to 10 days**

Fines are payable for late return

Speech Retarded and Deaf Children:

their psychological development

Edited by

Trian Fundudis, Israel Kolvin and Roger F. Garside

*Nuffield Psychology and Psychiatry Unit, Fleming Memorial Hospital,
Newcastle upon Tyne, England*

1979

ACADEMIC PRESS

London   New York   Toronto   Sydney   San Francisco

A Subsidiary of Harcourt Brace Jovanovich, Publishers

ACADEMIC PRESS INC. (LONDON) LTD.
24/28 Oval Road,
London NW1

United States Edition published by
ACADEMIC PRESS INC.
111 Fifth Avenue
New York, New York 10003

British Library Cataloguing in Publication Data
Speech retarded and deaf children.
1. Speech disorders in children – Great Britain
2. Child psychology
3. Children, Deaf – Great Britain
I. Fundudis, T
II. Kolvin, Israel   III. Garside, R
155.4'5'12   RJ496.S7   78-75264

ISBN 0–12–270150–x

Text set in 10/12 pt VIP Palatino, printed and bound
in Great Britain at The Pitman Press, Bath

Contributors

Editors

T. Fundudis, M.A., Ph.D., A.B.Ps.S. *Nuffield Psychology and Psychiatry Unit, Fleming Memorial Hospital, Great North Road, Newcastle upon Tyne NE2 3AX, England*

I. Kolvin, B.A., M.D., F.R.C. Psych., Dip. Psych. *Nuffield Psychology and Psychiatry Unit, Fleming Memorial Hospital, Great North Road, Newcastle Upon Tyne NE2 3AX, England*

R. F. Garside, B.Sc., Ph.D., F.B.Ps.S. *Nuffield Psychology and Psychiatry Unit, Fleming Memorial Hospital, Great North Road, Newcastle upon Tyne NE2 3AX, England*

Assistant editors

G. S. George, B.A. *35 Graham Road, Ipswich, Suffolk, England*

H. I. J. van der Spuy, M.A., Ph.D. *Department of Psychology, Chedoke Hospitals, Box 590 Hamilton, Ontario, Canada L8N 3L6*

Authors

P. Clarke, F.S.S. *Computer Division, Northern Regional Health Authority, Benfield Road, Walkergate, Newcastle upon Tyne, 6, England*

J. S. H. Nolan, M.A., M.Ed., A.B.Ps.S. *7 Osborne Avenue, Newcastle upon Tyne, NE2 1SQ, England*

E. Scanlon, L.C.S.T. *Fleming Memorial Hospital, Great North Road, Newcastle upon Tyne NE2 3AX, England*

L. G. Scarth, M.B.B.S., M.R.C. Psych., D.P.M. *Charles Burns Clinic, Queensbridge Road, Moseley, Birmingham B13 8QD, England*

E. G. Tweddle, B.A., R.G.N., S.C.M., H.V., R.N.T., C.C.P.N. *Fleming Memorial Hospital, Great North Road, Newcastle upon Tyne NE2 3AX, England*

R. M. Wrate, M.B.B.S., M.R.C. Psych. *The Young People's Unit, Tipperlin House, Tipperlin Road, Edinburgh EH10 5HF, Scotland*

Foreword

Since Sir James Spence created his astonishing service for children and their families, Newcastle upon Tyne has been the origin of many fundamental advances in our understanding of sick children and their families. This new book by Professor Issy Kolvin and his colleagues is worthy of that great tradition.

The work is firmly rooted in the real community of the north-east, and ascertainment covers the whole population. The study is prospective in nature. The enquiry is detailed with meticulous documentation of the early biography of each family. The copious data that have been collected are then analysed in a most sophisticated manner. This is a study without equal in the literature.

Speech disorders, both in the deaf and in those with good hearing, are a critical marker of deviant later development. The findings reported here have large implications for developmental screening and for remedial action in the pre-school years. They will be fundamental to the implementation of the Warnock Report.

The work deals with the whole range of deviant speech and language development. Infantile autism, elective mutism, dysphasia, dysarthria, deafness, hearing impairment, cerebral palsy and intellectual handicap are all individually surveyed. In addition a residual speech retarded group is identified. Its origins are described and analysed and its outcome is presented in detail.

This work is essential reading for all those concerned in child development.

April 1979   Christopher Ounsted

Human Development Research Unit
University of Oxford

Preface

Despite the burgeoning of interest in the language development of children, there have been relatively few studies that have attempted to address themselves to such a research theme from an epidemiological point of view. Futhermore, there have been even fewer which have combined the epidemiological cross-sectional with the longitudinal approach. Such approaches have been the tradition in Newcastle upon Tyne, as it was in this city that Dr Muriel Morley undertook her now classical study described in her book *The Development and Disorders of Speech in Childhood* (1957; second edition, 1965; third edition, 1972).

General practitioners, paediatricians, psychologists and psychiatrists are frequently confronted with questions from parents about the long-term consequences of delay in the development of speech and language in the early years of life. A commonly held view was that, provided that there were no associated major physical handicaps, most children would outgrow such problems so that, later, there would be no trace whatsoever of the previous delay. It was generally appreciated that greater precision was necessary, but this was bedevilled by insufficient information about the subsequent development of those children to allow clinicians to undertake reasonably accurate prognoses. Trained and experienced physicians were aware, for instance, that even among the speech delayed children who had no physical handicap, some had a less favourable prognosis than others, but it is important to know which type of speech-delayed children had the better prognosis. Furthermore, such views were based almost entirely on clinical impressions, as few studies had attempted to put such impressions into perspective by studying the subject at an epidemiological level. In addition it is essential to ascertain the relative importance of biological and psychological factors in relation to each other and to the environment, as a greater understanding of these factors and their relationships will aid prognoses and indicate the likelihood of response to particular forms of treatment.

There was, therefore, a strong case for studying a total population of speech retarded children prospectively, with particular emphasis on their subsequent performance in speech and language development, their intellectual development, their educational progress and their behavioural functioning. It was also essential to attempt to classify the disorders encompassed by the symptom of speech delay. It is hoped that the study will not only make a contribution to prognosis and classification, but also to the complex interrelations involved.

The book is subdivided into two sections. Part I is concerned with the speech retarded sample and comprises seven chapters. The first chapter describes the principles upon which we based the selection of our study population. The second chapter reviews the relevant literature on environmental and social factors. The next two chapters describe the results of the extensive and detailed series of assessments of the children's cognitive and behavioural development, carried out when the children were six, seven and eight years old. The following three chapters are devoted to clinical and statistical classification which try to define subcategories more precisely, and to ascertain the clustering and correlation of features in relation to these.

Part II is concerned with a hearing-impaired sample; it was considered to be important to include this because deaf children constitute a major group suffering from varying degrees of speech retardation. The deaf group was compared with the same control group that was used for research into speech retardation, and with the speech retarded sample itself. Chapter 8 defines the principles for selection of our deaf sample and also describes the findings relating to social and maternal factors. Chapter 9 briefly reviews the literature concerning cognitive and behavioural development of deaf children. The two remaining chapters concentrate on the intellectual and language development, educational progress, and assessments of behaviour and personality. The final Summary attempts to integrate the main findings of our research, covering both speech retarded and deaf children.

The scope of the research was so broad that it necessitated collaboration beyond our basic research team. We are, therefore, pleased to acknowledge the generous help of Mr Lionel Evans, Headmaster of the Northern Counties School for the Deaf and his staff; Mr A.S. Moore, organizer for partially-hearing units, Northumberland, and his colleagues; Dr K. F. Bailey, Deputy Director of Education; Dr L. F. Mills, Principal Educational Psychologist; Dr B. Shaw from the office of the Medical Officer of Health; and the Directors of Education and Medical Officers of Health over the period of the study, all of the city of Newcastle upon Tyne. We are grateful to the Heads of the Schools and their teaching staff who collaborated in rating the children's behaviour.

The study involved repeated examination of some 263 children over the early school years. The research depended entirely on the co-operation of the children and their mothers, and we are most grateful to them.

Indubitably the most important contribution from outside the research team was made by the late Dr Gerald Neligan. While he did not feel he had made a sufficient contribution to merit authorship of any of the chapters, this project was totally dependent on his generosity in relation to his Newcastle Child Development Study, which served as the source of material for our research. The editors received continued encouragement from Professor Sir Martin Roth and Professor Donald Court who were, at the time of the research, the respective Heads of the Departments of Psychological Medicine and of Paediatrics.

The research was originally planned by Professor I. Kolvin, Mrs Jane Nolan and Dr R. F. Garside. Mrs Nolan subsequently left the department and Dr H. I. J. van der Spuy and Dr T. Fundudis joined the team, later to be joined by Mrs Sandra George. The task of organizing the research, carrying it through its various stages, analysing the data and writing up the results was undertaken mainly by the three editors, who remained with the project throughout. Support was given to the editors by Dr H. I. J. van der Spuy and Mrs Sandra George. The major task of computer analysis was carried out by Mr P. Clarke, who is a member of the staff of Mr A. McNay, Statistician to the Newcastle Regional Health Authority.

A number of other collaborators were involved in various aspects of our research and, while it has not been possible to include them in this report, we nevertheless wish to express our indebtedness to them. They include the following: Mr J. W. Osselton, Senior Lecturer in Encephalography, University of Newcastle upon Tyne; Mrs Margaret Robson, Head Teacher, Nuffield Psychiatry Unit; Mrs Mary Harris, previously Head of Department of Speech Therapy, University of Newcastle upon Tyne and Mrs Dorothy Fisher (previously Muckle). Invaluable advice on audiometry was provided by Mr G. Chaytor, Regional Otologist; on method, by Dr T. T. S. Ingram of Edinburgh; Dr Michael Rodda and Professor R. Freeman critically reviewed the section on deaf children.

The research team is particularly indebted to Mrs Marjorie Blackburn, who conscientiously accepted responsibility for the administration of the research. Her efficiency and dedication was a major factor in enabling us to achieve a comprehensive assessment of the children and their families. She also accepted total secretarial responsibility.

Grants for the research were provided, initially by the Social Science Research Council, and subsequently by the Mental Health Research Fund.

April 1979 Trian Fundudis
Newcastle upon Tyne Israel Kolvin
Roger Garside

Contents

Part 1 A Study of Speech Retarded Children

1 Early development, types and prevalence
I. Kolvin, T. Fundudis and E. Scanlon

2 Speech retardation: environmental and social factors
G. S. George and I. Kolvin

xiv   Contents

3 A follow-up study: predictive importance—cognitive, language
and educational development
*T. Fundudis, R. F. Garside, H. I. J. van der Spuy, J. S. H. Nolan
and I. Kolvin*

4 Predictive importance—behaviour
I. Kolvin, T. Fundudis, G. S. George, R. M. Wrate and L. Scarth

Part II A Study of Hearing-impaired Children

8 The hearing-impaired child of primary school age: background factors, maternal attitudes and maternal personality
H. I. J. van der Spuy, T. Fundudis, I. Kolvin and E. G. Tweddle

9 Review of the literature: intellectual and language issues
T. Fundudis, I. Kolvin and R. F. Garside

10 The hearing-impaired child: intellectual and educational development
T. Fundudis, H. I. J. van der Spuy, R. F. Garside and I. Kolvin

11 The hearing-impaired child: behaviour and personality
I. Kolvin, H. I. J. van der Spuy, T. Fundudis, E. G. Tweddle and G. S. George

Part III Summary and Appendices

Summary
T. Fundudis, I. Kolvin, R. F. Garside

xviii · Contents

Part I
A Study of
Speech Retarded Children

1 Early development, types and prevalence

Introduction

There have been few systematic follow-up studies of children with speech retardation (Beckey, 1942; Morley, 1965; Fiedler *et al.*, 1971; Sheridan, 1973; Butler *et al.*, 1973). Even fewer have focused on a specific speech milestone and subsequently attempted to ascertain its usefulness as a 'screen' criterion or to study subsequent speech and other defects shown by the children who are retarded on this milestone. This was the main theme of the current follow-up which investigated children about seven years old who had shown speech retardation at the age of three. It has been pointed out (Butler *et al.*, 1973) that seven years is a convenient age for assessment of speech and language defects because by then most of the developmental mispronunciations have disappeared spontaneously, and those that remain are either intrinsically serious or have serious psychosocial implications.

Method

General

A survey (by Newcastle Child Development Study) of the entire population of children born in Newcastle upon Tyne provided an opportunity of studying longitudinally a full sample of speech retarded children. As part of the study, health visitors had recorded the developmental milestones of these children. We defined speech retardation as failure to use 'three or more words strung together to make some sort of sense' (Neligan and Prudham, 1969) by the age of 36 months. In this way a cohort of speech retarded children was identified. Admittedly *what was the background of examination?.*

this criterion is crude and arbitrary but it has the merit of being an objective, simple and standard way of recording developmental milestones. It is in fact a crude screening technique which has to be followed by intensive assessment and diagnosis. Using a total population sample avoids the selection bias which besets clinic and hospital studies. It also enabled us to study prevalence taking two factors into account:

(a) Although the size of the population (3300 children) was not large enough to produce reliable prevalence figures for relatively rare disorders, nevertheless, it provides a rough guide to the frequency of such disorders. *does it?*

(b) Using a symptom as an ascertainment criterion does not ensure complete coverage of the disorders which it identifies. This is because all children with such disorders do not necessarily have a speech delay of the severity defined by our criteria so that the prevalence figures reported provide only a conservative estimate.

Speech retarded sample

We decided to restrict the study to those children whose parents were still living in Newcastle when the child was aged three. Of the 133 thus identified from the Newcastle Maternity Study records we found that by the age of five years:

(a) 21 cases had left the area (15·7%);
(b) eight cases (6·1%) had to be excluded from detailed analysis because of inadequate or limited data because of hospitalization, being in care, twins (due to delayed computerization of twin records) or because parents refused to co-operate;
(c) two children had died (1·5%);
(d) there were 102 remaining children (76·5%).

Matched controls

The 102 remaining children were matched with normal controls on three criteria—age, sex and postal district. The matching was an administrative exercise utilizing population records. The subsequent assessments were undertaken 'blind'. However, in subsequent analyses involving comparison of subgroups with controls the individual matching was not maintained—the total control group was used for every comparison.

Testing

A series of psychological, educational and behavioural tests were administered (T.F.) which will be described later. In addition, speech and audiometric assessments (E.S.) and clinical assessments (I.K.) were undertaken. The mean age of the speech retarded group was seven years six months at the first psychological assessment and eight years four months at the second.

Diagnosis and classification (Table I)

The initial screen was essentially to identify children who were speech retarded. The subsequent diagnostic assessment at seven years identified those speech, language and other defects of which speech retardation is a symptom. This showed clearly that the cases could be divided into two broad groups.

, The *first group* consisted of those whose functioning, intellectually, psychologically or physically, was so abnormal that they were termed *pathological deviants*. Such cases fall into three relatively well-defined clinical groups and this is the basis of our operational classification.

(a) *Marked intellectual impairment* This was defined as an IQ at or below the 1st percentile on the WISC or where the child was untestable. In practical terms this means an IQ of 65 or below. This is possibly too rigorous a criterion as other authors have used a criterion of 2 standard deviations below the mean, i.e. an IQ of 70 or below (Yule and Rutter, 1970a).

(b) *Specific clinical syndromes* This included children with severe communicating disorders of childhood, such as elective mutism (Salfield, 1950; Brown *et al.*, 1963); infantile autism (Creak, 1961; Rutter, 1968, Kolvin *et al.*, 1971) and cleft palate/dysarthrias or severe language disorders.

(c) *Demonstrable neurological disorders* This includes children with cerebral palsy.

These categories were not intended to be mutually exclusive: some children showed features typical of all three categories, and were then classified according to the most predominant feature. Finally, we decided that deafness alone should not constitute sufficient grounds for labelling the child pathologically deviant.

The *second group* consisted of children who, after clinical examination at the age of seven, did not fall into the pathological category and hence have been described as the *Residual Speech Retarded Group*. More sophisticated psychological assessments were necessary to categorize the various characteristics of this group (Chapter 3).

The next problem was to reconcile this crude operational classification with a clinical classification of speech and language disorders. We decided to model our classification on the work of Ingram (1959 a,b, 1969, 1972). His is essentially a functional clinical classification and we have modified it both by abbreviation and simplification to suit our research as follows:

(a) *Dysarthria/cleft palate*—disorder of speech sound production with demonstrable dysfunction or structural abnormalities of tongue, lips, teeth or palate.

(b) *Secondary speech disorders*—disorder of speech sound production associated with other diseases or environmental factors:

    (i) mental defect
    (ii) hearing defect
    (iii) true dysphasia (acquired)
    (iv) adverse environmental factors
    (v) psychiatric disorders

Ingram (1972) points out that acquired dysphasia implies the loss of acquired language functions and so a birth-injured child cannot be described as having lost language functions, but more accurately as showing a retardation of speech development. In a child aged two to three years there is likely to be both impairment of language and thereafter slowing of speech development.

(c) *Specific developmental speech disorders*—the developmental speech disorder syndrome:

    (i) mild (dyslalia)
    (ii) moderate (developmental expressive dysphasia)
    (iii) severe (developmental receptive dysphasia, word deafness)
    (iv) very severe (auditory imperception, central deafness)

Ingram (1972) sees the developmental speech disorder syndrome as a descriptive label given to children with retardation of speech development, who are otherwise apparently normal in respect of their health, intelligence and home backgrounds. The features described by Ingram are: (i) apparently healthy children; (ii) average or superior intelligence; (iii) normal home backgrounds; (iv) high male–female ratio; (v) positive family history of slow speech development; (vi) an excess of ambidexterity and left-handedness in the first degree relatives; (vii) relatives who often have had difficulties in the early stages of learning to read and write (McCready, 1962; Brain, 1965).

In the past it has been assumed that, if a child has a unitary milestone delay and is in other ways not obviously abnormal, he will grow out of it. Such delays have been described by Rutter and Yule (1970) as representing 'extreme variations in normal development' which are 'related to the continuing growth and maturation of the brain'. Ingram, as described above, has stated what he considered to be the salient features of the developmental speech disorder syndrome. We consider that the following are some of the salient features of developmental delays (partly derived from Rutter): (i) they are more likely to occur in an isolated functional area rather than affect a wide range of milestones; (ii) they apparently are less likely to occur in younger children and children of lower mental age; (iii) they often occur where there is no evidence of structural abnormality of the brain; (iv) they tend to clear spontaneously as the child grows older; (v) boys are much more frequently affected than girls; and (vi) they may be influenced by environmental factors (Tizard, 1964).

Ingram (1972) points out that the label 'developmental speech disorder syndrome' is really a misnomer as the category comprises a heterogeneous group of articulatory and language disorders and in certain cases the speech development is not only retarded but is deviant as well. He finds it useful to regard this category as a spectrum of disorder which varies from the mild to the very severe. The mildest are the dyslalias which are defined as 'retardation of acquisition of word sounds but with normal language', i.e. the articulatory development of affected children is retarded. They are described by their parents as understanding the words but being unable to say them. Ingram also

Table I   *Classification and distribution by sex*

	Total	Male	Female
Category speech retarded	102	65	37
1 Pathologically Deviant	18	9	9
(A) Marked intellectual handicap			
(i) Subnormality mainly	7	4	3
(ii) Subnormality plus other conditions	13	7	6
(B) Cerebral palsy	5	3	2
(C) Specific syndrome			
(a) Autistic	2		2
(b) Electively mute	2	1	1
(c) Dysphasia	1	1	
(d) Cleft palate/dysarthria			
(i) Cleft palate/dysarthria alone	1		1
(ii) Cleft palate plus other conditions	2	1	1
2 Residual Speech Retarded	84	56	28

reports that the child substitutes or omits the later acquired consonants and consonant clusters inconsistently 'though his vocabulary and grammatical structures in spoken language may be within normal limits'. Children with moderate developmental speech disorders have normal comprehension but more severe retardation of word sound acquisition and retardation of development of spoken language. The severely affected children have greater degrees of retardation of word sound acquisition, impaired development of spoken language and impaired comprehension of speech. Synonyms for these three degrees of severity are 'dyslalias', developmental expressive dysphasia and developmental receptive dysphasia, respectively.

From Table I it will be seen that included in our pathological deviant category are Ingram's dysarthrias and secondary speech disorders. Our 'Residual Speech Retarded' Group comprised the remainder of the children and one could argue that these fall into the developmental speech disorder syndrome provided we widen Ingram's inclusive criteria to cover as well the dull range of intelligence and without stipulating a normal home background. It remains to be seen whether characteristic features of the syndrome can be indentified clinically or statistically.

Some background factors

Social class and speech retardation (Table II)

The breadwinner's occupation was coded in accordance with the Registrar General's Classification of Occupations (Great Britain, 1951). The speech retarded group's family social class tended to be lower than that of a random sample of Newcastle children (Neligan *et al.*, 1976). This is broadly in accord with the findings of other speech studies (Beckey, 1942; Morley, 1965; Butler *et al.*, 1973). However, as the control group in our study had been matched for postal district, we had expected that the controls and the speech retarded group would have had a similar distribution of social class; this was confirmed though the speech retarded group still showed a slight downward trend. The explanation which seems most plausible is that, even within urban areas or neighbourhoods, there is a relationship between child handicap and social class factors.

Sex differences

Rutter and Tizard (1970) report that there is a tendency for biological and perinatal hazards to occur more frequently among young males than females, with the inevitable consequence that a higher number of boys than girls are subsequently handicapped. This may be the basis for the greater vulnerability of boys to handicap, but is certainly not the whole answer (Ounsted and Taylor, 1972).

In most studies of developmental disorders, male:female ratios in the order of 2:1 to 3:1 are usually described. While the population sex ratio in Newcastle (1·04:1) approaches unity (Neligan et al., 1976) that of our speech retarded group was 1·7:1.

When the Residual Speech Retarded Group and the pathological deviants are analysed separately, the ratio is 2:1 for the former, and 1:1

Table II   *Social class distribution*

Social class	Controls (C)	Total speech retarded (T)	Residual speech retarded (R)	Random sample (RS)[a] $n = 208$
I + II	8 (7·9%)	5 (4·9%)	5 (5·7%)	9%
III	63 (61·8%)	53 (51·9%)	45 (53·5%)	61·0%
IV + V plus	31 (30·4%)	44 (43%)	34 (40·2%)	29·5%
Total	102 (100% approx.)	102 (100% approx.)	84 (100%)	(100%)
Statistic Chi-squared		C vs T = 3·81 2 d.f: NS	C vs R − 2·1 2 d.f: NS	T vs RS = 6·1 2 d.f. $p < 0.05$ R vs RS = 3·4 2 d.f. NS

NS = Not Significant
[a] From Neligan et al. (1976)

for the latter. This leads to the preliminary conclusion that the sex ratio of the former group resembles that described in developmental disorders.

We wondered whether there would be any change in the sex ratio in the Speech Retarded Group if we took into account whether they were early or late walkers and we found that the ratios were 1·7:1 and 2·1:1 respectively. In other words, the ratio does not change substantially when we separately analyse early and late walking speech retarded children.

In brief, as already described, separate analysis of the pathological deviant group and of the Residual Speech Retarded Group gave male:female ratios of 1:1 and 2:1 respectively, suggesting that the high male:female ratios reported in the literature (Butler et al., 1973) are probably more related to developmental delays than to disorders with an organic basis.

Milestones and the specificity of speech retardation

The other signs of developmental retardation are of considerable import. We were anxious to find out whether the milestone delay in children in the Residual Speech Retarded Group was specific to speech or general in nature.

There are a number of ways of tackling the above question but we confined ourselves to attempting to identify a group of children with speech delay which was not associated with a delay in beginning to walk.

As previously stated, our criterion for speech retardation was failure in using three-word sentences by 36 months. This corresponds to the 97th percentile based on Neligan and Prudham's (1969) norms for developmental milestones (based on the total population of births in Newcastle upon Tyne over a three-year period). We defined walking retardation as walking later than the 90th percentile (using Neligan and Prudham's norms)* which in practice meant grouping of children according to whether they were walking before or after 16 months. A child was therefore considered to have a general delay in milestone achievement if he was retarded in speech and in addition had not walked unsupported by 16 months. Next, we identified a group of children who were retarded in speech but walked early, i.e. had a specific speech delay. For this purpose early walking was defined as walking at or below the 25th percentile (according to Neligan and Prudham's norms), i.e. at or before 12 months. The above method identified three groups:

(a) Specific speech delay, i.e. a group of 25 children who walked early but were speech retarded. Using the above criteria the minimal rate is about eight per 1000 children.
(b) An intermediate group of 34 (who were speech retarded but walked by 16 months).
(c) General milestone delay, i.e. a group of 23 children who walked late and also were speech retarded. Using the above criteria the minimal rate is again about eight per 1000 children.

---

* Neligan and Prudham's percentile norms are presented in reverse of the more usual form; the 97th percentile would, therefore, presumably have read as the 3rd percentile, and so on, in the more customary form.

Two children who proved to be deaf were excluded from this classification (see p. 16 and Chapter 3).

Other milestones

From Table IIIa it will be seen that the Residual Speech Retarded Group achieved bladder control and unsupported walking later than the controls, but this was statistically significant for walking only. However, it will be noted that these statistics do not take into consideration the

Table IIIa   *Milestones—three-year-old data*

	Controls	Residual speech retarded	Pathological deviant	Control *vs* RSR group
Bladder dry by day n =	94	72	7	
m (in months)	23·8	25·8		NS
s.d.	5·9	5·8		
Not yet dry n =	8	12	11	
Walking unsupported n =	102	84	10	[a]
m (in months)	13·4	14·5		
s.d.	2·1	3·7		
Not walking n =	0	0	8	

[a]$p < 0.01$.

higher percentage of the Residual Speech Retarded (14%) who were not yet dry by day at three years of age compared to the controls (8%). While the mean age of walking of the controls is close to Neligan and Prudham's (1969) 50th percentile, that of the speech retarded group is closer to their 75th percentile level. This means that our Residual Speech Retarded Group is, on average, less retarded in walking than in speech. Some may interpret these findings as reflecting uneven maturation while others may interpret them as an expected regression to the mean. Further, it will be noted that the pathological deviants' other milestone development (bladder control) is seriously retarded.

Laterality

Faulty cerebral dominance has been implicated as the basis of developmental language disorders (Orton, 1937, 1934). However, in a recent survey of the literature (Rutter and Yule, 1970a), it was found that reports of excess of left and/or mixed laterality in speech retarded children tend to be highly contradictory with 'as many reports of negative findings as of positive findings'. This is, of course, to be expected in that most of the previous studies have been clinic or hospital ones. The same is true of studies of reading retarded children where high rates of left or mixed-handedness have not been found even when the study was epidemiological rather than hospital-based (Belmont and Birch, 1965; Douglas *et al.*, 1967; Rutter and Yule, 1970a).

The current research provided further opportunities for studying such questions. As shown in Table IIIb, there are no significant differences in

Table IIIb   *Dominance and laterality at age of eight*

	Controls	Residual speech retarded
Hand preference (Harris)		
Right dominance	68%	62%
Hand–foot dominance		
discrepancy	52%	51%
Hand–eye dominance		
discrepancy	40%	49%
Left–right differentiation difficulty	19% (19 out of 99)	37%[b]

[b]*p* <0·01.

terms of right, mixed or left-handedness between the controls and the Residual Speech Retarded Group; nor were there any significant differences in the number of right, mixed or left-eyed children between the groups. The only significant differences concerned the ability to differentiate between the right and left sides of the body; the speech retarded children were significantly worse in this respect (*p* < 0·01). This important finding is re-examined in relation to intellectual developments in Chapter 3. These somewhat surprising findings provide unequivocal evidence that an unselected sample of children with delayed speech development show no more left hand or eye preference or inconsistencies of preference (mixed handedness or eyedness) than the normal population. It remains to be seen whether different types of classification may lead to the emergence of associations which have been masked by the lack of conceptualization. This question is examined in subsequent chapters.

Perinatal factors

The mean gestational ages of the pathological deviant group and also the Residual Speech Retarded Group were significantly shorter than that of the controls. This finding is similar to that described by Butler *et al*. (1973) in children with speech defects. However, unlike the Butler study, we did find significant differences in birth weight between our total speech retarded group and the controls. The only other perinatal index which revealed differences was that of the second stage of labour which proved significantly longer in our total speech retarded group than the controls.

Birth order

Fewer of the speech retarded children were first-born. While this achieves statistical significance (Table IV) the absolute figures are not as

Table IV   *Sibling order*

Position	Controls		Residual Speech Retarded Group	
	n	*%*	*n*	*%*
Eldest/only	35	35	15	19
2nd or 3rd	41	41	48	57
4th or 5th	20	20	14	17
6th or more	6	6	7	9

Significance–Chi-squared = 8·0, 3 d.f, p <0·05.

impressive as in the National Child Development Study (Butler *et al.*, 1973). On the other hand, the mean family size reveals a trend for the Residual Speech Retarded to come from larger families (mean of Residual Speech Retarded Group = 4·35; of controls = 3·37).

Prevalence findings

We have already noted that 31 of the original 133 cases were not available for full testing at school age. Such losses constitute a potential source of bias and hence it is important to know how far the fully tested group can be regarded as representative of the total cases identified as being retarded in speech at the age of three years. Fortunately, information gathered in the perinatal period and in the first five years of life was contained in the records of the Newcastle Child Development Study (Neligan *et al.*, 1974). We confined ourselves to checking basic characteristics where fuller information was likely to be available. The characteristics chosen were occupational social class of breadwinner and the rate of serious handicap in the children. The distribution of the occupational social class of the families of these 31 children proved to be slightly better and the rate of serious handicap no greater than in the group available for assessment (with the exception of the two children who had died). We therefore concluded that those children who were not seen were unlikely to differ significantly from those assessed at school age.

When calculating prevalence rates it is necessary to make appropriate adjustment for such losses. Our formula for this consists of multiplying the rate of disorder by a factor of 1·30.

Prevalence of speech retardation at the age of three

At the age of three years some 4% (133) of 3300 children had retardation of speech reported by health visitors. This is a lower percentage than that described in the 1000 family study (Spence *et al.*, 1954; Morley, 1965) where a 6% retardation is described at the same age using broadly similar criteria in a random sample of 114 children. However, it is likely that these slight differences can be accounted for both in terms of the definitions of incomplete sentences (simpler in our study) and the fact that the data in the 1000 family study was derived from an examination by speech therapists. It is of importance to note that in the 1000 family study about 1% were still using incomplete sentences just before starting school.

Disorders at follow-up: prevalence and comment

Of the 102 speech retarded children studied at the age of seven, 18 (17·6%) fell into the pathological deviant category. The subcategories in Table I are not intended to be mutually exclusive and hence the sum of the frequencies in these is greater than the total number of cases.

(a) Pathological deviants

(i) *Infantile autism*   A rate of two to four per 10,000 children has been described by Lotter (1966) in his Middlesex survey. Our rate of 0·8 per 1000 is broadly consistent with Lotter's rate. This is of considerable importance as there has been some speculation about whether the rate reported by Lotter is only applicable to the more affluent southern areas of England. The above figures suggest this rate is true for both the north and the south and for both affluent and industrial areas of the country.

(ii) *Elective mutism* We recorded only two 'nuclear' electively mute children (Tramer, 1934) with an inordinate and selective shyness of strangers severe enough to persist into the seventh year of life. Browne (1963) feels that elective mutism is more common than is generally believed. However, the frequency is dependent on whether it is broadly or narrowly conceived and defined. Indeed, norms for shyness relative to age would enable a clearer distinction to be made between unusual shyness which occurs frequently in the pre-school period (Kolvin and Nolan, 1978) and the pathological shyness which occurs in elective mutism. We have used the latter, more narrow definition and therefore consider 0·8 per 1000 as a minimum prevalence rate particularly as there remains the theoretical possibility that electively mute children could have slipped through our screen at the three-year-old stage. Appropriate enquiries were made to ascertain if any cases had been referred to colleagues, both for the purpose of this study and a specific study of elective mutism (Kolvin and Fundudis, 1979) but no further cases were uncovered. Elective mutism would therefore appear to be as rare a syndrome as infantile autism.

(iii) *Dysphasia* Similar problems of definition confound frequency and prevalence studies of childhoold dysphasias. Some use both verbal behaviour and presumed aetiology as criteria whereas others use verbal behaviour alone (Ingram and Reid, 1956; Morley, 1965; Lenneberg, 1967; Eisenson, 1968). Even though one can theoretically make the distinction between an acquired dysphasia (Ingram, 1972) and the moderate or severe form of the specific developmental speech disorder syndrome (Ingram, 1972), which some would label as developmental expressive or developmental receptive dysphasia respectively, in practice we found the distinction difficult because of the partly retrospective nature of the diagnostic exercise. In fact, we uncovered only one case which could be included in the clear-cut severe dysphasic category. This represents a rate of 0·4 per 1000 children. The prevalence of serious and persisting language disorder has been estimated as approximately 0·7 per 1000 in Scotland (Ingram, 1963) at the age of five, and 0·8 per 1000 on the Isle of Wight (Rutter *et al.*, 1970a). MacKeith and Rutter (1972) point out that there are no reliable figures for persistent disorders involving a defect in language comprehension, and estimate that the rate is very much less than that for infantile autism. Our figures support the suggestion that the condition is as rare or even rarer than infantile autism.

(iv) *Cleft palate/Dysarthria* Morley (1965) reports one case of cleft palate per 1000 births and we found two which represents a rate of 0·8 per 1000.

(v) *Deafness, hearing impairment* Deafness is one of the major causes of delay in language development (Morley, 1965). It has been estimated (Pless and Graham, 1970) that about two per 1000 children have deafness severe enough to merit the use of hearing aids. But the rate in the case of profound deafness is even lower than this. The latter estimate is supported by our own two cases with profound hearing loss—a rate of 0·8 per 1000. Additionally another two, though not profoundly deaf, were in special educational settings for children with multiple handicaps. This leads to a rate similar to those reported by Barton et al., (1962), Reed (1970) and Neligan et al. (1974) in the major Newcastle survey of which this study forms a part. (As the two cases presenting with profound deafness and language retardation showed only minimal signs of other handicaps we decided for the purposes of this study not to include them in the pathological deviant group in our subsequent analyses.)

We defined hearing impairment as hearing loss of 20 decibels or more on at least four out of the seven frequencies tested in each ear. Any loss of less than 20 decibels was considered to be within the normal range, provided that there was no high frequency loss. Details of audiometric assessments are presented in Chapter 5. Hearing loss of 20 decibels or more occurred in 15% of the 80 children in the Residual Speech Retarded Group, which is not significantly higher than the controls where it occurred at a 9% rate. This is, however, double the rate reported by Anderson (1967) but we do not consider the findings of these two studies comparable because of the different definitions. Such rates are predictably lower in a survey than in clinic populations—for instance, Morley (1965) reported that over one-third of 280 children referred to her with delayed speech development had 'insufficient hearing'.

(vi) *Cerebral palsy* The cerebral palsy rate (Mackeith and Rutter, 1972) is two to three per 1000 (Ingram, 1955; Rutter et al., 1970). If cases with severe intellectual handicaps are excluded the rate falls to one per 1000 who have, in addition, language retardation. Our rate for a combination of cerebral palsy and speech and possible language retardation is about 2·0 per 1000. This closely approximates the rate reported by Neligan et al. (1974) in the major survey of which our study forms a part.

(vii) *Intellectual handicap* The single most common cause of slow speech development in paediatric clinics is mental handicap (Ingram, 1972). Ingram points out that this is to be expected as it has been shown in a number of studies (Illingworth, 1966) that while motor milestone in a significant proportion of intellectually handicapped children may be within normal limits 'milestones of speech, adaptive and social behaviour development are invariably achieved late. But even so the degree of retardation of speech development is not always proportional to the severity of mental defect in later life.' Finally, Ingram (1972) points out that intellectually handicapped children tend to have a high degree of environmental deprivation and a conspicuous proportion of hearing defects compared to children of average intelligence.

The rate of handicap is dependent on the definition employed. Rutter et al. (1970a) defined it as an IQ of less than 70, and reported that over $2\frac{1}{2}$% have intellectual handicap and that over half of these show severe language impairment or articulation defects or both. Our criterion was more rigorous, i.e. an IQ of 65 or below (1st percentile or below) using the WISC performance norms. We decided to use these norms because it was considered invalid to use a verbal criterion in a group of speech retarded children. When we included cases of autism and cerebral palsy who have severe intellectual handicap, we found that some 13 children had both severe intellectual handicap and speech retardation. The rate, therefore, is about 5·1 in 1000. If we employ the criterion of a performance IQ of 70 or less then the numbers marginally increase to 14 and the rate becomes 5·5 per 1000. An analysis of our data (see Chapter 3) reveals that if we had used the full scale IQ as a criterion the picture would have dramatically changed. The use of the performance IQ as a criterion was based on clinical experience where at times it can be demonstrated that some children with poor speech and language abilities can function better on non-verbal tests (Rutter, 1972). Research on autistic children (Rutter and Lockyer, 1967) has provided evidence of the predictive importance of performance tests. However, Rutter (1972) points out that such findings need to be validated on other language disordered populations.

(b) The Residual Speech Retarded Group and its relationship to the developmental speech disorder syndrome

It will be remembered that these comprise the remainder of the children who did not fall into the category of being 'pathologically deviant'. If we make no qualification about intelligence or home background (provided we exclude children with severe intellectual handicap) these children could be considered as falling into Ingram's specific developmental speech disorder syndrome. The prevalence rate is then in the vicinity of 3% of children of school age.

Questions still remain about the severity of the disorder: how many children are mildly affected, having retardation of acquisition of word sounds, but with normal language (dyslalias), and how many children are severely affected, with retarded spoken language development (dysphasias). Such difficulties are underlined by Mittler (1970), who points out that there is considerable disagreement about the difference between 'the mere late development of language and some kind of specific developmental disorders of the dysphasic type'. Further, language comprehension normally precedes language production (Fraser *et al.*, 1963; Lovell and Dixon, 1967) which leads mothers of even normally developing children to comment that their children can understand a great deal before they can speak. By the same token, children with developmental disorders may have a normal understanding of language before they can talk (Lenneberg, 1962). From clinical experience this is particularly true of the 'dyslalias' and developmental expressive dysphasias where, in the latter, the discrepancies can be particularly marked. Obviously such discrepancies, though helpful in diagnosis, can hardly be considered specific to the dysphasias.

Clearly, diagnosis undertaken after the age of seven cannot easily identify which children were dyslalic and which dysphasic, as the disorders mostly correct themselves (Morley, 1965). However, more sophisticated psychological testing theoretically could reveal a cluster of cases with a pattern similar to that obtained with dysphasic children (Olson, 1961). This will be the subject of a subsequent chapter.

Fluency and articulatory ability at the age of seven

Disorders of word sound production can occur in the dysarthrias, with defective sensory input, and in the developmental speech disorder syndrome. We studied articulation using the Edinburgh articulation test, which led to quantitative assessments of the child's articulatory skills. (In consultation with Mr Pellowe, of the Linguistic Department of the University of Newcastle upon Tyne, we modified the test slightly to accommodate local dialectical variation.) This test (Anthony, 1971) provides norms only up to the age of $5\frac{3}{4}$ years. Obviously such norms are not applicable to our children. On the other hand, it appeared reasonable to use this test as a means of obtaining standardized measures of articulation for comparison of age-matched groups of children. In Table Va it will be seen that the Residual Speech Retarded Group have a significantly lower mean score of correct items than the controls. The incorrect items were further analysed using a modification of Anthony's (1971) qualitative assessment system. She describes five categories of errors and we have varied this using the following three categories only: (a) almost mature; (b) immature (including very immature); and (c) atypical substitutions. The atypical errors were rather infrequent in both groups, but the most striking example of it occurred in the one pathological deviant case who was diagnosed as being clearly dysphasic. As shown in Table Va the mean number of immature errors was significantly greater for the speech retarded group. From Table Vb, which provides a distribution analysis of these immature errors, it can be seen that some 70% of the speech retarded group (as compared to 35% of the controls) had six or more immature errors. These findings again emphasize the importance of following up the total sample of children to ascertain their later speech development.

Table Va *Assessment of speech at seven years using Edinburgh articulation test*

		Controls (n = 100)	Residual speech retarded (n = 80)	Statistical significance
Correct score	m	59·5	52·5	$p < 0.01$
	s.d.	8·6	12·4	
Immature errors of articulation	m	4·9	9·9	$p < 0.01$
	s.d.	6·2	7·6	

Table Vb *Distribution immature errors of articulation*

Range	Controls		Residual speech retarded	
0–5	65	(65%)	24	(30%)
6–14	26	(26%)	40	(50%)
15+	9	(9%)	16	(20%)

Sig. Chi-squared = 21·9, 2 d.f., $p < 0.01$

Using the Andrews and Harris scale (1964) we found one mild stammer in each group. Andrews and Harris' work suggested that about 3–4% of children of school age stammered for a period, but in only about 1% of children was this more persistent. Our findings appear to be in accord with the latter figure as our assessment of stammer was based on a conversation with a child at one point in time. There is a suggestion in the literature (Andrews and Harris, 1964; Ingram, 1972) that stammering is more common in children who have been delayed in language development. As our sample was rather small it is difficult to be absolutely sure, but it does not provide evidence that stammering is more common in children who have previously been speech retarded.

Concluding comments

Our results emphasize the predictive value of a simple speech screen at the age of three years. About one in five of the 4% of all children aged three years who were speech retarded were later found to have serious language, intellectual or physical handicaps. It is also important to note that almost half of these handicapped children were found to be functioning rather poorly in what appeared to be inappropriate educational settings. This underlines the value of an early screening exercise (Butler *et al.*, 1973) in identifying children with handicaps who need help, for both accurate diagnosis and appropriate placement. Such a screening procedure could be applied quite easily by a health visitor or a general practitioner who could then refer the identified children to the appropriate paediatric clinic. Findings from the national study (Butler *et al.*, 1973) support the view that it would be preferable to institute screening procedures before the age of seven.

Some might argue that screening at the age of three years would pick out too many 'false positives', comprising subsequently spontaneously remitting cases of developmental speech delay. However, as yet, there is inadequate information about how this group of children function intellectually, educationally, behaviourally and socially at older ages. This is the subject of later chapters in the book. What must be emphasized is that what happens at three does not reflect the total position at five, six or seven years, so that a comprehensive screening programme should include periodic re-screening over the first five to seven years of life.

We have put forward arguments to support the theory that the Residual Speech Retarded Group can be considered as falling into the developmental speech disorder category. However, while the distribution of certain factors, such as the sex ratio, support this view, othejs, such as laterality, do not. Further, it is evident that even if most cases can be, by a *tour de force*, included in a so-called developmental speech disorder category, this category is clearly heterogeneous (Ingram, 1972). For instance, our research has demonstrated that there are at least two subgroups—one with general delay of milestones and one with a specific delay of speech. In a subsequent chapter we examine the profile of features found in the above subgroups and those reported in the literature which contribute to the syndrome of developmental dysphasia.

Finally, we have to consider the influence of adverse environmental factors (McCarthy, 1954; Bernstein, 1961, 1962). We have not, in fact, tried to separate a group of children suffering from sociocultural retardation, mainly because such a procedure implies that once a group of children has been separated environmental influences subsequently do not adversely affect the remaining children. We believe instead that there is a continuum of adverse environmental factors; in a subsequent chapter we will attempt to quantify these factors and to compare their frequency in our speech retarded group with our control group.

2 Speech retardation: environmental and social factors

Introduction

The purpose of this chapter is to describe information obtained in a series of interviews with the mothers of speech retarded children. These interviews had a dual aim; first, to obtain information on the behaviour of the children (this information is incorporated in Chapter 4 and therefore will not be described further in this account), and, second, to obtain a broad descriptive picture of each child's environmental background and, in so doing, to investigate certain specific hypotheses.

The main hypothesis embracing this part of the investigation was that environmental factors affect the acquisition and early development of speech and language. For the purpose of this study 'environment' was seen as the present and past family and social background of the child, covering basic demographic factors and such variables as the amount of appropriate stimulation in the home, the attitude and expectations of the parents, especially the mother, the stability of the home and so on. It was thought that such factors were likely to be of as much importance in the development of speech of children with physical handicaps as they would be to the child not suffering from any gross disorder.

Review of literature relating to effects of environmental variables on the acquisition of speech

It is a common view that 'Man is born to talk' (Hebb *et al.*, 1971) and the present-day preoccupation with language is an acknowledgement that it is the pivot of man as a social and thinking being. The child who is deprived of the richness, flexiblity and creativity of speech as a means of communication is indeed severely handicapped, and the conundrum of why a 'normal' child, surrounded by spoken and written language from birth, fails to develop a competence which is so essential to him is a matter of considerable interest. The contribution of environmental factors to speech and language development is a matter of controversy as are the reasons for the failure of these children to acquire speech normally. While theorizing currently widely exceeds empirical knowledge, some of the major theories have nevertheless generated valuable hypotheses capable of being scientifically tested.

In the past two decades the part played by environmental factors in the acquisition of speech has been played down on theoretical grounds by Chomsky. In 1957, Chomsky, who has emerged as one of the most creative linguists of this century, published a controversial article in opposition to the extreme empiricism of B. F. Skinner's *Verbal Behaviour* (1957). In this classic book, Skinner, by conceiving language as yet another learned skill, acquired by means of simple stimulus–response conditioning, inevitably placed the onus of successful learning upon environmental factors. Chomsky rejected the behaviouristic standpoint in relation to language development, stating, 'What evidence is now available supports the view that all human languages show deep-seated properties of organisation and structure. These properties—these linguistic universals—can be plausibly assumed to be an innate specific mechanism, a 'language-acquisition device' (LAD), which determines the structure of language' (Chomsky, 1965). The relevance of such complex and far-reaching theories to the problems of delay in the acquisition of speech is that delay must consequently be viewed as having a basis in structural, neurological deficit.

Lenneberg (1966) gives credence to this theory by adding neurological and observational support. He argues persuasively that the emergence of speech is most easily accounted for by maturational changes which are amazingly unaffected by abnormal factors in the child's environment, and which are independent of practice or needs. He and others have pointed out that children of deaf parents were found to babble appropriately and to develop speech adequately even though brought up in a grossly abnormal linguistic environment. Comparative studies of normal and defective children have shown speech development to be remarkably synchronized with motor milestones, and Lenneberg states, 'The preservation of synchrony between motor and speech or language milestones is, I believe, the most cogent evidence that language acquisition is regulated by maturational phenomena.' Morley's (1965) findings, in her classic longitudinal study of speech development, support this view by failing to find any association between adverse social factors, such as the mother's ability to cope and the child's failure to learn to talk.

The extent of the swing from the extreme behaviourist position to that of the extreme nativists would itself suggest the acceptability of a middle-ground position, and theories acknowledging the interaction of innate and environmental characteristics are persuasive on common-sense grounds. According to Piaget, for example, the development of language is dependent upon diverse cognitive abilities which have arisen in the sensori-motor period (the first two years of life) as a result of the infant's innate tendency to exercise his reflexes and to organize his actions as a response to the need to adapt to the environment. It is essentially a theory of accretion, as is that of Bruner and his associates (1969), whose detailed studies have well illustrated the essentiality of the interaction between the child's innate behaviours such as seeing and pointing behaviours, and the mother-figures' responses. Bruner describes the extremism of Chomsky and Skinner as 'a miraculous theory on the one side and an impossible theory on the other'.

Similarly, Hebb et al. (1971) demolished the claims of extreme nativists by proposing 'a more moderate view in which learning cooperates with heredity in the child's mastery of language'. He states,

'We believe that how learning occurs, and what learning, is as much determined by the learner's heredity as by his environment. In behaviour that
depends on perception and thought, the relation of constitution to experience
is multiplicative rather than additive; to ask what is more important is like
asking which contributes more to the area of a field—its length or its breadth.
Both are of 100 per cent importance, even when one is a greater source of
variance than the other, and their relation is such that one must understand
both to understand either.'

His own theory stresses the importance of latent learning, involving perceptual learning (Gibson and Gibson, 1955), sensory pre-conditioning in which the association between two stimuli is learned by their being simultaneous (Brogden, 1947) and one trial learning. 'Latent learning without reinforcement is one of the facts of human behaviour, a normal consequence of perception.'

These cursory indications of the theories of Piaget, Bruner and Hebb are perhaps sufficient to show that, although essentially very different, they nevertheless have in common a stress on the interaction between heredity and environmental factors, and thus justify an examination of the impact of environmental factors and human communication.

Indeed, weighing up the evidence, it is unlikely that narrow extreme theories will prove to have more than moderate validity. Wider multi-factor theories are likely to explain much more than single factor theories (Werry, 1972; Kolvin et al., 1973b). For instance, theories taking into consideration the relationship between intrinsic (biological) factors and extrinsic factors such as learning, social and psychological factors, are likely to be more credible and to have greater predictive validity. An examination of extrinsic influences upon the development of speech therefore is justified, though always bearing in mind the likelihood of such factors being tempered by their interaction with intrinsic factors. Taking an analogy from the theory of bladder control (Kolvin and Taunch, 1973), a mature biological substrate implies the potential for control of wetting but not necessarily the presence of control and needs to be complemented by an experiential or learning component. Such control can fequently be accelerated by the use of a conditioning technique. With regard to speech and language functioning two allied questions have to be tackled: first, can specific training and general enrichment or stimulation accelerate the rate of maturation of the biological substrate, leading to earlier vocalization, earlier onset of meaningful speech and quantitatively better syntactic and semantic development? Second, once the biological substrate is mature, can specific training and general enrichment in stimulation lead to significant, syntactical, semantic and cognitive gains; and, if so, can these gains be maintained?

The evidence so far suggests that certain speech milestones are relatively independent of environmental influences. First, there is the onset of babbling even in the case of congenitally deaf children; second, there are only small social class differences in relation to the age at which children start to speak (see Chapter 1); and, finally, aspects of early language development of slum children as compared with controls do not appear to be significantly retarded (especially with regard to syntactic development). Even small differences may be called into question as they may partly be determined by cognitive and not social class effects alone.

It has been shown that the development of certain aspects of language ability in earlier years is sensitive to the amount and nature of the interaction of the child with parent figures (Ainsworth and Bell, 1974; Beckwith, 1971; Rheingold, 1960). This will be discussed later. If we narrow the field to vocal development, there is evidence that prebabbling behaviour seemingly related to later vocal development is susceptible to environmental stimulation. Trevarthen et al. (1975) showed, by analysing films of mother–baby interactions, that very young babies made specific mouth movements in response to their mothers' voices and, perhaps equally important, the mothers spontaneously imitated with vocalizations the movements of their infants' mouths.

There are numerous studies, comprehensively summarized by Rutter and Mittler (1972), which have shown that after babbling begins appropriate verbal and social reinforcements tend to increase the amount of vocalization (Todd and Palmer, 1968). Verbal enrichment with continuous reinforcement increases not only the quantity but also the type of vocalization (Routh, 1969; Rutter and Mittler, 1972). The importance of social interaction at this stage is underlined by Lenneberg's findings (1966) that, in deaf children, babbling develops at the normal age and continues for some time, but then begins to fade because of the lack of auditory stimulation. It is more likely to continue if the deaf child is able to see the adult who is speaking to him. (Rutter and Mittler, however, warn against the presumption that there is a necessary connection between babbling and later language development.)

We are therefore left with the question concerning whether general stimulation and specific training can significantly enhance syntactic, semantic and cognitive development. Some preliminary findings by Brown and Hanlon (1970) suggest that mothers in their children's early years are more likely to reinforce semantic and phonetic components of speech and language than to correct sentence construction. On the other hand, specific attempts to achieve syntactic correctness by repeating the child's utterances in a syntactically correct manner prove less effective than varied and informative interchange between parent and the child (Cazden, 1966; Brown et al., 1969). The fact that attempts to 'reinforce' syntactic correctness have proved to be more effective than no training at all suggest that combinations of syntactic and semantic training are likely to have the best outcome. Such work is still in its early stages with workers exploring the use of such techniques to facilitate syntactic development (Jeffree, 1971). However, in real life, middle class mothers are likely to provide their children with appropriate syntactic and semantic experience and, by the spontaneous use of social reinforcers, to condition appropriate responses.

Though there is obvious importance in a two-way verbal exchange after the emergence of true speech, the actual way in which learning occurs is by no means obvious. The role of such commonly accepted mechanisms as imitation is not clear-cut. Rutter and Mittler (1972) argue that 'imitation provides only a minor direct influence on syntactical development. However, it may well be more important in the learning of vocabulary or in articulation.' Nevertheless, children do imitate what is said to them, and Brown and Bellugi (1964) found that adults, too, in speaking to children simplify their speech and imitate the child's form of utterance. Imitation, too, can be viewed as a form of conditioning using the operant paradigm.

Studies of institutionalized children have thrown light upon the importance of appropriate verbal enrichment and stimulation and social reinforcement. Rheingold (1961) found that infants in institutions did not suffer in their development or social responsiveness up to about three months of age. Provence and Lipton (1962) indicated, however, that thereafter such infants quickly become less alert and less responsive. Goldfarb (1943) studied the language of children who spent their first three years in an institution, comparing their subsequent development with that of children who spent their first three years in foster homes. The children were tested throughout childhood and into adolescence, and the orphanage children were found to be retarded linguistically and also failed to progress beyond very low levels of conceptual activity.

It has also been found that insufficiency of stimulation, as with prolonged institutional experience (Haywood, 1967; Lipton, 1969), has adverse effects on language development and verbal intelligence even in infancy (Brodbeck and Irwin, 1946; Provence and Lipton, 1962). Such adverse effects of insufficient stimulation are not confined to institutions but are demonstrable even with children living with their families where there is grossly inadequate verbal stimulation (Jones, 1954). In their penetrating analysis, Rutter and Mittler (1972) therefore emphasize quality of care (Haywood, 1967; Tizard, 1969) rather than whether or not the child remains at home with parents. For instance, in institutions where the quality of care is good there is little in the way of adverse effects (Yarrow, 1964; Tizard, 1971) and similarly Kibbutzim children are not affected (Kohen-Raz, 1968). It has now also become clear that a constant background of noise of people speaking is less than an optimum experience for language development. It is the quality of adult–child interactions (Rheingold, 1960, 1961) which is important either in the home or in an instituion. A number of authors suggest that, in institutions, where there is a constant background of noise, it becomes difficult to distinguish relevant foreground stimuli from irrelevant background ones (Spradlin, 1968; Rutter and Mittler, 1972; Mittler, 1972). Such an explanation is supported by the finding of poorer verbal intelligence and vocabulary scores of children in large families (Douglas, 1964; Douglas et al., 1968). Many workers agree (Douglas et al., 1968; Rutter and Mittler, 1972) that the most likely explanation is that the elementary grammar and vocabulary of the pre-school child pro-vides insufficient stimulation to other children, compared with adult–child interactions. However, another way of explaining this phenomenon is that it is not the richness (and often irrelevant noise) of environmental stimulation but rather the clarity and quality of the adult–child interactions that are important (Friedlander, 1971; Rutter and Mittler, 1972).

The above considerations are particularly well illustrated in working class families. Furthermore, working class school children show inferior language performance (Templin, 1957; Lawton, 1968), vocabulary know-ledge and verbal intelligence (Douglas et al., 1968). As already discus-sed, social class influences appear to be selective, as the differences are small in relation to certain speech and language milestones, but are broad in relation to language usage and educational performance. Rutter and Mittler (1972) point out that such differences are less marked in relation to language competence and more marked in relation to abstract language functions and the way in which the latter are used.

The question now arises as to the type of mechanisms by which such enhanced abstract language functioning is achieved. Specificity appears to be important, as middle class mothers are more specific and informative in talking to their children and answering questions, and middle class children are more specific in their language usage than in the case of the working class (Hess and Shipman, 1965; Rackstraw and Robinson, 1967; Brandis and Henderson, 1970).

These aspects have been elaborated by Bernstein (1958) who described differences in language usage when comparing middle class children with working class children. Bernstein distinguished different forms of communication codes—*public*, later called *restricted*, which is mainly used by the working classes, and *formal*, later called *elaborated*, which is mainly used by the middle classes. Some workers have interpreted Bernstein's concept in terms of a clear-cut distinction between the codes, but such an absolute distinction was never intended. Indeed, it is best thought of as a continuum which at its elaborated end is characterized by a wide syntactical repertoire which is used to express ideas, and in complex grammatical sentences of good syntactical construction, with a wide use of adverbs and adjectives and a varied and flexible use of conjunctions, and so on. The understanding of a statement in restricted code is often dependent upon the knowledge of the listener, the use of non-verbal communication, such as gesture, and the social context in which it is used. There is evidence to indicate that general usage of the restricted code does not indicate that the speaker is totally unable to use the elaborated code, but that the potential for usage of certain aspects of the elaborated code is retained to be used in certain limited situations (Robinson, 1965). However, incorporated in the theory is the implication that insufficient use of the elaborated code could impair its development.

So far our discussion has confined itself to the development of language and verbal intelligence. For the sake of completeness some comment on cognitive development is needed. While the influence of certain institutional experiences and social class effects is particularly important to the development of vocabulary and higher order language functions involving abstraction and conceptualization, non-verbal cognitive behaviour is less affected by such influences. Furthermore, the well-known association of verbal IQ and family size does not hold to the same extent for performance IQ. Thus performance IQ appears to be relatively independent of such environmental influences.

In the USA theories stressing social class differences in language and cognitive development were given formal recognition and financial support with the inauguration of the massive State-supported Head-Start Programme. In a rush of ideological enthusiasm, compensatory language programmes were designed nationwide for the 'culturally deprived child'. Initially, results seemed to show unbelievable gains in the children's linguistic and cognitive abilities, and euphoria reigned. Cultural and environmental influences had apparently at last been confirmed as important agents in a child's mastery of language and the development of his cognitive abilities. But the euphoria was short-lived. Long-term follow-up assessments showed that the intellectual gains dissipated if nothing more was done for the child. However, some of the better programmes which had involved the parents or the elementary school did report more durable IQ and language gains, so the pendulum was not allowed to swing right back to pure nativism. Instead it was recognized that children's cognitive abilities were not entirely plastic but that, nevertheless, within certain limits their abilities could be improved by appropriate stimulation as long as this was continued. As a result, Parent–Child Development Centres have been set up by the State Officer of Child Development where the emphasis is more upon educating the parent to be an educator rather than directly stimulating the child. It is too early for firm conclusions but there are indications that such mother-directed intervention has more durable effects upon the child's competence.

Conclusions

There is compelling evidence that environmental factors influence vocal abilities, from babbling to the mastery of adult speech, and that deprivation leads to less than full achievement of potential. But can any real-life situations be so devoid of appropriate stimulation that the 'normal' child, the subject of our original problem, is, as a result, slow to acquire speech, regardless of how far that speech might be from what we regard as most culturally acceptable? Everyday observations would lead us to question this assumption. The middle class mother might provide the 'required' stimulation by involving her child more in one-to-one conversations, reading to her child and so on, but the working class child is frequently immersed in the greater stimulation of the hurly-burly of life in larger families, where the mother is less isolated from her friends and relatives, and where, perhaps, the father participates more in verbal exchanges because of the flexibility of his employment pattern or indeed because of his unemployment. Any research project involving home visits to children from different social backgrounds leads one to question which background is, in fact, the most 'deprived'. Labov (1970) underlines the illogicality of the view that lower class children come from verbally deprived backgrounds, saying of the research in such areas:

'We see a child battered in verbal stimulation from morning to night. We see many speech events which depend upon the competitive exhibition of verbal skills: singing, acting and oratory—a whole range of activities in which the individual gains status through his use of language. Even though we might accept that speech patterns vary with social class, the concept of "verbal deprivation" is subtle and complex, and creates class-barriers.'

Accordingly, in the research described here attempts were made, which proved only partially successful, to control for social class in order that such environmental influences, and hence differences, would be kept to a minimum (see Chapter 3).

Method

The interviews were carried out with the mothers. Where there was no mother at home because of death or separation (four cases) then basic 'hard' information was obtained from the father or parent substitute, but naturally all mother-dependent ratings such as those concerned with mother's attitudes, relationship between mother and child and assessments of mother's speech were inapplicable in these cases. (As this was well under 5% of our data we considered that our analysis was in no way invalidated.)

Initial communication with each family was by a letter which introduced the study by explaining that we were attempting to investigate the development of a random group of children, and that someone would call to see them to explain the nature of the research with a view to enlisting their co-operation. In this subsequent visit our interest in child development in general was explained but no mention was made of any particular interest in speech. As all of these families remembered that their children had been studied in the first few years of life as part of the 1962 Newcastle Child Development Study, it seemed logical that there should be a follow-up of their children at about seven years of age. Face-to-face contact reduced initial anxiety and eventually most families co-operated fully (see Chapter 1).

An important part of the research design was that the interviews were conducted blind; the interviewer did not know at the time of interview to which group a child belonged, this information being solely in the hands of the organizing secretary. Nevertheless, it usually became apparent early in the interview whether or not the child belonged to the pathologically deviant group, but it was rarely apparent whether or not he came from the Residual Speech Retarded Group or the control group. After the major part of the environmental, attitudinal and maternal speech information had been collected, general questions about the early development of the child and finally his speech development were asked. It is interesting to note that, in subsequent analysis, it was found that almost half of the parents in the Residual Speech Retarded Group denied any delay in their child's acquisition of speech, whereas 14% of the control group did think that their child had had a speech disorder. Thus, the mothers' memory lapses lessened possible control versus experimental bias in ratings.

The first interview consisted wholly of semi-structured open-ended questions: the data to be collected was clearly specified and the method of questioning was partially specified; nevertheless the interviewer was allowed to diverge from the formal layout at her discretion. The areas covered comprised:

1 Basic demographic, descriptive data of the family, and also detailed measures of such features as interaction between child and mother, and intellectual activities in the home.
2 An assessment of the child's emotional behaviour and temperamental characteristics by means of a behaviour (Kolvin et al., 1975) and a temperament questionnaire (Garside et al., 1975).
3 An assessment of the mother's speech by means of a strict quantitative analysis and, in addition, a subjective assessment by the interviewer.
4 Assessment of mother's sociability by means of the Wallin's Neighbourliness scale (1954).
5 Assessment of the mother's reported behaviour in disciplining situations and when answering the child's questions, by means of a technique developed by Robinson and Rackstraw (1967) and Robinson (1969).

The second interview was similarly semi-structured and consisted of the collection of further demographic and descriptive data of the family and child; in addition, at the end of the interview the following questionnaires and tests were administered:

1 The Eysenck Personality Inventory (1964)
2 The Maryland parental Attitude Questionnaire (Pumroy, 1966)

In assessing the contribution of social, family and other environmental factors to the acquisition of speech we were faced with the problem of the complexity of the relationship between the variables studied. We examined a large number of features, many of which appeared to contribute towards a small number of broad themes. In such circumstances we decided to sum the measures to provide an index of the particular adverse factor (theme) under consideration, arbitrarily giving the constituent variables equal weighting. This was achieved by studying the distribution of scores on a particular measure, deciding on an extreme cut-off, and a score above the extreme was given a weighting of 1 for that measure. There are obvious advantages in summing scores which appear to be meaningfully related. First, the summed score will be more reliable than its constituent variables, and second, it greatly simplified the analysis and hence the description of the findings. Such summed scores are referred to in the text as indices.

A different aspect of the problem of analysis was the probable multiplicative rather than purely additive relationship between some of the background factors and outcome. This is considered elsewhere in this book (Chapter 7).

Findings

1 Perinatal and developmental factors

Perinatal risk index

Ten extreme perinatal obstetric experiences or complications were all given equal weightings (of 1). These were summed to give the 'perinatal risk index'. These included such factors as antenatal complications, toxaemia of pregnancy, complications of delivery, foetal distress, etc. There were no significant differences between the three groups studied. The constituent items were also studied but few significant differences were found.

Early infancy illness score (Table I)

This was an index of illness leading to hospitalization, infectious disorders, fits, convulsions, etc. All these were given equal weighting (of 1) but meningitis or encephalitis were given a double weighting (of 2). This is, in fact, a non-specific type of illness index. There were no significant differences between the controls and the Residual Speech Retarded Group, but a highly significant difference between controls and pathological deviants. This indicates that some of these illnesses are likely to be of aetiological significance in the case of a subgroup of the pathological deviant group.

An analysis of the constituent items revealed that the only individual item for which there were significant differences between the groups was the higher incidence of convulsions amongst the pathological deviant group.

Developmental difficulties index (Table I)

This was a measure based on developmental delays of the child in areas other than speech. Evident difficulties or delays in sucking, swallowing,

Table I   *Indices of adverse physical, development or environmental factors*

	a = Controls	b = RSR[a]	c = PD[b]	Significance 5%	1%
(a) *Development difficulties index score*					
families with index of 0	69	45	3	a *vs* c	
families with index of 1	25	26	8		
families with index of 2 or more	7	9	7		
(b) *Early infancy illness score*					
families with index of 0	51	37	9		a *vs* c
families with index of 1	29	29	2		
families with index of 2 or more	22	15	7		
(c) *History of speech disorder*					
families with index of 0	88	49	14		a *vs* b
families with index of 1	12	27	3		
families with index of 2 or more	2	7	1		
(d) *Family developmental risk index*					
families with index of 0	88	51	11		a *vs* b
families with index of 1	12	22	7	a *vs* c	
families with index of 2 or more	2	7	0		
(e) *Adverse family experience index*					
families with index of 0	58	33	5	a *vs* b	a *vs* c
families with index of 1	23	22	2		
families with index of 2	12	14	5		
families with index of 3 or more	9	11	6		
(f) *Structural defects of language*					
families with index of 0	79	50	9	a *vs* b	
families with index of 1	19	22	6		
families with index of 2	3	5	1		
(g) *Language literacy index of mother*					
families with index of 0	37	14	1	a *vs* b	
families with index of 1	32	27	7		
families with index of 2	28	29	7		
families with index of 3 or more	3	7	1		
(h) *Social environment risk index: risk score*					
families with index of 0	40	17	1		a *vs* b
families with index of 1	33	20	3		a *vs* c
families with index of 2	14	14	7		
families with index of 3 or more	15	30	6		
Maximum *n* =	102	83	18		

[a] RSR = Residual Speech Retarded Group
[b] PD = Pathological deviant group

taking solids and walking were each again given equal weightings. These were summated to give the developmental difficulties score. The only significant difference was between the pathological deviant group and the controls. A study of the constituent items revealed that only the pathological deviant group showed significant differences on some of these as compared with the control group.

Summary

The Residual Speech Retarded Group did not differ in any way from the controls either in terms of perinatal experiences or early physical development. As expected, there were many significant differences between the controls and the pathological deviant group.

2 Evidence of developmental difficulties in the family (Table I)

Family developmental risk index

Historical evidence of developmental speech delays in either parent was given a weighting of 1; with a similar weighting for evidence in sibs. Left-handedness in either parent was given a weighting of 1, and again, left-handedness in any sib was given a similar weighting. The maximum score per case was therefore 4 and the minimum 0. It will be seen that there is a very evident excess of such characteristics in the Residual Speech Retarded Group.

Family history of speech disorders

This was an index of historical evidence of speech disorder. We requested information about delays in speech development and stutters or stammers. If parents provided affirmative evidence in the case of mother, father or any sibling then the family was given a weighting of 1 for each of the two disorders. Thus the theoretical maximum score for a family was 6. There was a highly significant excess of such disorders in the Residual Speech Retarded Group as compared with the controls.

Summary

Members of the families of children in the Residual Speech Retarded Group clearly have suffered from more developmental difficulties than were found in families of control children.

3 Social factors

Social class

Social class was rated for each family according to the breadwinner's occupation, or last occupation if not currently employed. As has previously been described (Chapter 1) in matching the speech retarded children with controls an attempt had been made to control for social class by selecting children from the same areas of the city. In spite of this, however, the speech retarded children showed a downward social class gradient compared to the controls, but this did not prove to be significant (see also Chapter 3). Other aspects of social disadvantages were also studied.

The social·environmental risk index (see Table I)

The social/environmental risk index was obtained, by summating weighted scores on the following items:

   (i) Type of housing
  (ii) State of home
 (iii) Person/room ratio
 (iv) Number of children born to mother (5+ children = 1)
  (v) Poor work record of breadwinner
 (vi) Mother working when child three years old
(vii) Contact with social agencies

There was a highly significant difference between the control group and both criterion groups, denoting an excess of social inadequacy in both the latter groups. Six of the seven constitutent items in this index were significant in their own right and merit further analysis.

Housing (see Table II)

The 'state of the home' item was designed to assess the quality of cleanliness, order and repair in the home, and, as such was a reflection of the family's ability or inability to cope. The homes of children in both speech retarded groups were in a very significantly poorer condition than were the homes of the controls. There was also significantly more overcrowding in the houses of both speech retarded groups. Finally, the mothers in these groups had significantly more children.

Work patterns of parents (see Table II)

Fathers in both speech retarded groups were more likely to have unsatisfactory work patterns when compared with those in the control

Table II *Social factors*

	a = Control group	b = Residual Speech Retarded Group	c = Pathological deviant group	Statistical test	Significance 5%	Significance 1%
State of home						
good	80	48	9	chi-squared		a vs b
fair or poor	20	34	9			a vs c
Person/room ratio—mean	1·04	1·19	1·31	t-test	a vs b	a vs c
No. of children born to mother—mean	3·37	4·35	4·75	t-test	a vs c	a vs b
Work pattern of father						
satisfactory	72	48	5	chi-squared	a vs b	a vs c
unsatisfactory	30	36	13		(almost)	
Mother working when child 3 years old						
no	92	65	15	chi-squared	a vs b	a vs c
yes	10	16	3		(almost)	
Mother working when child 8 years old						
no	60	55	8	chi-squared		a vs c
yes	42	26	9			
Contact with social agencies						
no	95	63	13	chi-squared	a vs c	a vs b
yes	7	19	4			

Control group $n = 102$ (reduces to 100 for certain comparisons).
Residual Speech Retarded Group $n = 84$ (reduces to 81 for certain comparisons).
Pathological deviant group $n = 18$ (reduces to 17 for certain comparisons).

group. The global rating of unsatisfactory work pattern was defined as the breadwinner having lost at least two months' work in the last year due to illness, unemployment or malingering, or having changed jobs at least three times in an occupation where this is not likely to be acceptable. The fathers in the pathological deviant group had a significant excess of unsatisfactory work patterns. Though there was a similar trend for the fathers in the Residual Speech Retarded Group, the difference did not quite reach significance levels.

There was a tendency for more mothers in both speech retarded groups to work during their children's pre-school years (RSR almost significant at $p = 0.05$; PD $p <0.01$). It is interesting to note that this trend was not continued, and that by the time the child was eight years old a greater percentage of mothers in the control group were working than mothers in the Residual Speech Retarded Group, though *not more* than in the pathological deviant group. The difference, however, was not quite significant. Many explanations, all speculative, can be offered for such findings. Perhaps in the Residual Speech Retarded Group there were early pressing economic needs for the mothers to work, whereas the control group mothers' return to work could be postponed to a more convenient time, such as when the children were at school. At this time the control group mothers were *more* able to take advantage of the work opportunities than the Residual Speech Retarded Group, perhaps because there was less likelihood of younger children being in the home. Once again, in the work pattern of both parents in the early years, the speech retarded groups are seen as being in a socially disadvantageous position. Later we offer an alternative explanation for the high percentage of mothers of the pathological deviant group going to work when their children were of school age.

Contact with social agencies (see Table II)

This rating was designed to assess the number of contacts the family had with various social agencies in the year prior to the child's birth, the assumption being that inability to cope with social problems would result in a greater than average number of contacts. (This information had been collected at birth as part of the Newcastle Child Development Study—Neligan *et al.*, 1974.) Contact with the following agencies was counted: National Assistance Board; Probation Service; National Society for Prevention of Cruelty to Children; Women's Voluntary Service; Red Cross; Church Social Services; School Welfare Officer; Citizen's Advice Bureau. Both speech retarded groups had a significantly higher number of contacts with social agencies, a clear indication that these families were already subject to increased social stresses at the time of the child's birth.

Summary

Despite attempts to control occupational social class differences between groups by matching the control group with the speech retarded groups in terms of the local neighbourhood (postal district) we found that according to occupational social class ratings (Registrar General) there was still a trend towards a downward gradient of the two study groups compared with the controls (see Chapter 1). We have previously advanced the hypothesis that even within the same urban area or neighbourhood there is a relationship between social factors and child handicap. Occupational social class, however, is a relatively crude index of social disorganization or malaise. We consider our social environment risk index a more sensitive measure for assessing or reflecting adverse social enviromental factors. Indeed, on this index significant differences were found, with both speech retarded groups having higher risk scores than the controls. In common with findings in similar investigations of other handicapped groups, these social factor differences were compounded of a multitude of social problems and poorer coping ability as shown by impaired employment patterns, poor housing and increased contacts with social agencies. In conclusion, our attempts to control for social class factors were only partially successful; such factors, therefore, cannot be totally discounted when interpreting our various findings.

4 Psychological tensions and stress in the home

The adverse family experience index (Table I)

This was a summated score which was intended to indicate the amount of emotional and behavioural disturbance within the home during the child's lifetime. It was composed of weightings of items (using the same method as before) which indicated stress or poor coping behaviour of individual members of the family. Such items included poor sociability of the mothers; the total length of separation of the child from its mother; the child living with neither parent; the civil state of the parents; whether the parents had ever separated; any psychiatric treatment of the father, the mother or the siblings and stress during pregnancy. On this summated score the families in both speech retarded groups showed significantly more evidence of psychological stress. An analysis of the constituent items reveals the following.

Sociability of mother A self-rating inventory (Wallin, 1954) assessed the amount of social contact that the mother enjoyed; mothers in both speech retarded groups showed a tendency to be less sociable than the mothers in the control group.

Separation of child from parents While all the control group children lived with at least one of their parents at the time of interview, four of the children belonging to the Residual Speech Retarded Group were not living with either parent. Furthermore, there was a trend for children in the Residual Speech Retarded Group to have been separated from their mothers for a greater length of time in the first five years of life than had the control children. It was not valid to draw comparisons with the pathological deviant group because of the greater likelihood of these children having been in an institution.

Civil state of parents and separation of parents There was no difference between the groups in relation to marital state, but there was suggestive evidence of marital tension in the two speech retarded groups in that there was a tendency for the parents of these children to have experienced more temporary separation as the result of marital conflicts.

Psychiatric treatment of family members Information was obtained about psychiatric treatment given to fathers, mothers and siblings. Only with regard to the mothers were there any interesting differences between the groups. There was a tendency for the mothers in both speech retarded groups to report that they had received more help of a psychiatric nature during pregnancy than had the mothers of the control group, and this was particularly marked for mothers in the pathological deviant group (Table III). Subsequently, there was a similar tendency for mothers in both speech retarded groups to seek help from their family doctor for more minor psychological problems and, again, this occurred more frequently in the case of the pathological deviant group (but the differences were not statistically significant). Information was also obtained from the mothers about more serious psychological problems meriting attendance at psychiatric clinics subsequent to the birth of the child; the pattern contrasts markedly with the above picture—in no instance did a mother from the pathological deviant group report attendance at such a clinic whereas ten of the mothers of the Residual Speech Retarded Group had done so (Table III).

The interpretation of these findings is made difficult by the interaction of the stress caused by caring for a handicapped child with the stresses related to adverse social factors. Nevertheless, we consider that the higher rates of more minor psychological problems reported by mothers in both the study groups is likely to be related to their socially disadvantageous backgrounds. A similar explanation can be offered for the high rates of the more serious psychological problems reported by the mothers in the Residual Speech Retarded Group. However, if psychiatric disturbance is brought on or exacerbated by the additional burden of caring for a handicapped child, we would have predicted that the mothers of the pathological

Table III *Psychological background factors in relation to mothers*

	a = Control	b = Residual Speech Retarded Group	c = Pathological deviant group	Statistical test	Significance 5%	Significance 1%
Mothers attending psychiatric departments						
no	100	70	18	chi-squared		a vs b
yes	2	10	0			
Psychiatric disorder in pregnancy						
no	87	64	12	chi-squared	a vs c	
yes	14	16	6			
Social disturbances in first year after birth						
no	95	65	15	chi-squared		a vs b
yes	7	16	3			
Time before mother felt back to normal self (in months)	8·99	16·99	18·78	t-test	a vs b	
Mother's reading index						
no	36	44	Not applicable	chi-squared		a vs b
yes	65	37				
Assessment of mother's speech						
adequate	98	72	13	chi-squared		a vs b
inadequate	4	9	3			

Control group maximum $n = 102$.
RSR maximum $n = 84$ (reduces to 80 for certain comparisons).
PD maximum $n = 18$ (reduces to 16 for certain comparisons).

deviant group would have been more likely to be in need of treatment from a psychiatrist than would mothers of the Residual Speech Retarded Group. This was not so, however, and we can only speculate as to the reasons. From Table II it will be noted that more of the mothers of the pathological deviant group were working when the children were of school age, despite the severity of handicap of their children. Clearly this was facilitated by the day or residential/institutional care made available to their children. We can only suggest that this work experience may have had a moderating influence on the emotional stress which results from having to cope with a seriously handicapped child.

It is also difficult to know what to make of the findings of the differences of psychiatric disturbance in pregnancy, described above, because of the tendency of certain mothers of seriously handicapped children to provide distorted accounts of perinatal experiences—almost as if they were looking for something in their pregnancy which could have been responsible for their child's disorder.

Two related scores, which were not included in the social environment risk index, throw more light upon the social factor which might have affected the mother's psychological state. First, mothers were questioned about any disturbing factors in the environment in the first year of the child's life which might have been expected to have had a deleterious effect upon the relationship between mother and child. The factors considered were any events which might reasonably have been expected to affect the psychological well-being of the mother, such as violence in the home, acute financial difficulties, death or severe illness in the family, though factors which were directly attributable to the psychiatric state of the mother herself were naturally not counted. The Residual Speech Retarded Group suffered significantly more social disturbances than the control group (Table III).

The second score was simply a count of the length of time in months before each mother felt that she was back to her normal self again after the birth of her child. The mothers in both speech retarded groups tended to take longer, but the difference was only significant for the Residual Speech Retarded Group. Whilst such a finding is to be expected, perhaps, in relation to the mothers in the pathological deviant group, who had to cope with the stress of an often severely handicapped child, the significance of the finding in the Residual Speech Retarded Group, taken in conjunction with our findings relating to disturbance in the first years of life, would suggest increased tension and stress which was not directly attributable to factors within the child himself. Such stress, we feel, might reasonably have been expected to have led to impairment in the mother's maternal role, but this is purely speculative.

Summary

There was more evidence of tension and stress in the families of both speech retarded groups which manifested itself in a tendency to increased temporary marital separations, significant increased social disturbance in the first year of the child's life and also in minor psychological disturbance of the mothers. Though the mothers of the children in the pathological deviant group might well have been expected to be under increased psychological stress because of the severity of their children's handicap, such an explanation would seem to be insufficient to account for the fact that the mothers of children in the Residual Speech Retarded Group showed equivalent levels of minor psychological disturbance when their children's handicaps were, in the main, so much less severe. It seems reasonable to assume that the disturbances in the latter group were less likely to be attributable to the child's handicap, but were more a reflection of tensions associated with the greater loadings of adverse social factors already described. Furthermore, despite the social and psychological burdens which the mothers of the pathological deviant children had to carry, not one had described the presence of more serious psychological disturbance. We offer the explanation that opportunities for special schooling or care, giving rise to greater opportunities for work, constitute protective influences.

5 Speech, language, literacy and social factors

Innumerable studies have shown that the language abilities of the child who has already acquired speech can be influenced by environmental verbal stimulation. In this study an attempt was made to investigate whether the acquisition of speech can be affected in a similar manner. Various assessments were made of the quality of the verbal/literacy stimulation which the children currently received, working on the assumption that this is likely to reflect the level of verbal stimulation which the child received in the early years of its life when speech is normally acquired.

Quantitative assessment of mother's speech

Tape recordings were made of the interviews with the mothers. Though the greater part of the interview was semi-structured, mothers were at one point asked four set questions. Their replies to these four questions were subjected to a detailed quantitative grammatical analysis similar to the Templin/McCarthy system we used in the assessment of children's speech, with modification suggested by the work of Hess and Shipman (1965). (A more detailed account is availabe from S.G.).

It was originally intended to rate the total replies to the four set questions. However, as the system we used involved a straight count of various categories of parts of speech, a simple quantitative analysis might give a higher, and hence better, score to a more garrulous response, and a lower score to a precise, clear and brief response. We therefore had two alternatives. The first was to rate the response not only qualitatively but quantitatively as well. The second was to prune redundant words, which are those used in falters of fluency, stammers, unnecessary repetitions and unfinished sentences, and then to assess the first 100 non-redundant words. When less than 100 non-redundant words were used in reply to the four set problems, then the mother's reply to questions in another specified section were included. The above decision proved to be correct, as length of utterance correlated inversely with sentence complexity.

The analysis fell roughly into three areas. First, there was a straight count of the number of words which fell into various grammatical categories, such as verbs, nouns, prepositions, co-ordinating conjunctions, subordinate conjunctions, etc. In children's speech such quantification gives an indication of the structural complexity and hence the maturity of the individual child's speech. It was assumed that this would apply to adult speech, too. However, whilst the scores in a few grammatical categories did appear to differentiate slightly between the groups, the differences were not significant and at times proved to be in opposite, inconsistent directions. The second procedure involved scores of complexity derived from an analysis of the clause and phrase structures of the sentences, but again these failed to differentiate between the groups.

Whether our failure to find differences between the groups with these first two techniques was due to a lack of sensitivity of the assessment instruments or to a real lack of differences between the groups is difficult to say. One could hypothesize that if there had been a familial tendency to delayed speech, this was likely to improve spontaneously with maturation and hence the negative result. On the other hand, Hess and Shipman did report that this kind of analysis differentiated successfully between adults from different social groups. However, we may have been expecting more from this crude approach than it could really achieve. It needs to be emphasized that there were no between-group social class differences measured in the traditional way. In other words, the social discrepancies between the various groups studied may not have been sufficiently great (compared to those encountered by Hess and Shipman) for any differences to emerge.

Structural defects of language (Table I)

Whatever may have been the reason, syntactical quantification did not succeed in reflecting differences between these groups and it was decided, therefore, to concentrate mainly on our third group of categories, which were those designed to measure 'errors' of speech. These were combined into a cumulative index which we named 'structural defects of language'. This was composed of the following sub-categories:

(i) Incomprehensible sentences. These were sentences which were nonsensical either in structure or in subject matter, or were rendered meaningless by their being grossly unintelligible. Two or more of such sentences were given an adverse score of weighting of 1.

(ii) Total number of redundant words. Redundant words were those which hindered the clear expression of the mother's thought and fell into the following categories: falters in fluency; stammers; verbal tics and unfinished sentences. A score of 20 or more redundant words was given an adverse weighting of 1.

(iii) Total number of grammatical errors. This was a simple count of grammatical errors, and two or more were given an adverse weighting of 1.

(iv) Total number of incomplete sentences. These were sentences which were both structurally and functionally incomplete. (A sentence which is not structurally complete can nevertheless be seen as functionally complete if it is meaningful in the context of the sentence spoken before or after by the speaker himself or by the interviewer.) Two or more functionally incomplete sentences were given an adverse weighting of 1.

The distribution of scores of the three groups on this index is shown in Table I, where it is seen that the mothers of the children in the Residual Speech Retarded Group had a significantly higher structural defect score than had the control group. The distribution of scores of the mothers of the pathological deviant group suggested that there might be differences, but the sample size was too small to allow such differences to emerge. Analysis of the sub-categories themselves showed that the mothers of the two speech retarded groups consistently scored less than the controls, but the differences were not always significant.

Language literacy index of mothers (Table I)

This was a broad category covering the types of experiences which theoretically could directly or indirectly influence the child's speech and language development. It included six items covering literacy, reading, assessment of the mother's speech, grammar and syntax. There were significant differences between the mothers of the controls and the Residual Speech Retarded Group. There were also differences between the groups on some of the constituent items.

(i) *Mother's reading index* (Table III) This was an assessment of the number of times a mother spent listening to her child read (only those children at home). It was originally intended to be a rating of the number of sessions the mother spent reading with her child in the last typical week, but so many mothers failed to read at all with their children that a simple dichotomous rating of whether or not the mother read with her child at least once per week was substituted. The mothers of the Residual Speech Retarded Group were significantly less likely to read with their children, even though the nature of the child's reading handicap would mean that he would be less likely to read by himself without help from his mother. We would have expected, therefore, an increased index rather than the reverse, but in fact 54% of the mothers failed to read with their children. This finding could be interpreted as due to either the mother's lack of appreciation of and concern for the child's needs, or due to the child's unwillingness to read. Either way, the child most in need of help actually received less.

(ii) *Mother's literacy* We assessed the mother's literacy by simply recording whether the mothers could read sufficiently well to complete proformas such as the Maryland Attitude Questionnaire, etc. with little or no help, or whether the proformas had to be read out to them for completion. Ten mothers in the Residual Speech Retarded Group and two in the pathological deviant groups needed help. Again, this may just reflect the weight of adverse social circumstances or poorer social origins of these mothers.

(iii) *Assessment of mother's speech* (Table III) The interviewer made a subjective judgement as to whether the mother had adequate or impoverished speech. Impoverished speech was defined as having limited use of vocabulary, reliance on intonation and gesture, short incomplete utterances, constant recourse to useless interjections, and a repetitive use of words resulting in a marked overall difficulty in conveying meaning and in understanding questions. (The reliability was assessed by two independent ratings of a sample of 20 speech extracts and a correlation of 0·74 was achieved.) There was a non-significant excess of mothers with impoverished speech in the Residual Speech Retarded Group. However, the absolute numbers are not impressive.

Summary

While quantitative assessment of mother's speech revealed no major differences between the groups, assessment of structural defects of language did reveal differences. Our results demonstrated that the mothers in both speech retarded groups were more likely to be deficient in speech and literacy.

Again, it is difficult to interpret these findings. They may reflect the loadings of adverse social factors present in families in the two experimental groups. Alternatively, they may represent a syndrome of minimal impairment of speech and language present in a subgroup of the Residual Speech Retarded Group; the features of such a syndrome could be the residual sequel of a more evident but spontaneously resolving speech retardation which has a familial basis. It is important to note that these differences are not readily observable and only become evident when relevant constituent items are summed to produce an index of a structural defect of language.

In addition to assessing the verbal stimulation received from the mother directly, we measured other environmental factors which might have influenced the child's verbal ability. These were:

(i) Presence of television in the home
(ii) Television programme watched
(iii) Regular newspapers and magazines purchased
(iv) Child's membership of library
(v) Child's purchase of comics

Not one of these variables significantly differentiated between the Residual Speech Retarded Group and the controls. Although the last two variables did differentiate between the pathological deviant group and the control group, this was of no significance because of the severity of the children's handicaps.

Nursery school

Various studies (e.g. Randall *et al.*, 1974) have indicated that attendance at nursery school has a marked beneficial effect on language development. In this study no differences were found between the Residual Speech Retarded Group and the controls in terms of attending Local Authority nursery schools or private nursery schools.

Speech therapy and elocution lessons

It was surprising that very few children had remedial speech help. No child had elocution lessons. One child in the control group had speech therapy (lasting at least two months), but 11 in the Residual Speech Retarded Group and four in the pathological deviant group did so as well.

Mother's strategies in disciplining and their ways of coping with their children's questions

An analysis was undertaken of the content of mother's speech when faced with situations requiring explanations, as when they answered their children's questions, or responded to their children's misdemeanours. This followed closely the very detailed and extensive studies undertaken by Robinson, Cook and Rackstraw (Robinson, 1969), which had as their impetus the theories of Bernstein mentioned earlier. Briefly, mothers in the study were asked how they would reply to various set questions if they were asked by their children. Their answers were analysed in terms of accuracy, and type and amount of information made available to the child. In addition they were asked what they would say to their children in six situtations in which they might consider the child in need of discipline. Different modes of action they could take were analysed (e.g. physical punishment, verbal punishment, avoidance of action, reparative acts, supportive strategies). A detailed analysis was also made of the reasons given to the child for the necessity of changing his behaviour. (For a full account of this analysis the reader is referred to the original papers by Robinson, Cook and Rackstraw (Robinson, 1969) or to the present authors.)

This data was analysed in various ways—in terms of differences between groups on individual items, summations of similar items and by principal component analyses. While some differences were in the expected direction, few significant meaningful differences emerged between the groups. In brief, mothers in the two criterion groups were less likely to give meaningful comprehensive answers to questions and were more likely to discipline without explanation. However, as the differences were small we are of the opinion that they can be discounted, as they were unlikely to make any significant contribution to the children's poor speech development. The reasons for the lack of importance of such factors in our study is probably the result of matching for neighbourhood and hence cultural factors. The slight increase of negative strategies which we found in our criterion groups are probably related to the social class gradient which in fact was not statistically significant.

Conclusions

We have demonstrated the importance of the contribution of perinatal factors and early infancy illness factors in relation to the pathological deviant group. On the other hand, a family history of developmental delays occurred more frequently in the case of the Residual Speech Retarded Group and this confirms an often reported association. This gives rise to the hypothesis that there may be a familial developmental component in at least a subgroup of the Residual Speech Retarded Group.

Despite controlling for social class a significant excess of adverse social factors was found in both study groups. This is probably a manifestation of the fact that even within the same neighbourhood there is a gradient of social factors, with a tendency to a clustering of adverse social experiences where there is demonstrable evidence of child handicap.

Quantitative grammatical and syntactical analyses of mothers' speech revealed no significant difference between the groups. However, there was a significant excess of developmental speech delays and associated problems in the families of the study groups but the distribution of such problems in the control group is unexpectedly high.

Again, the language literacy index, which can be considered a measure of the cultural-educational stimulation, reveals the presence of less of such stimulation in the Residual Speech Retarded Group. We have already postulated that this finding is simply a reflection of the slightly lower social class distribution of the study groups. It is interesting to note that this social class gradient is not reflected in the mothers' coping and disciplining strategies. We again suggest that an even steeper social class gradient may be necessary for such differences to emerge.

We advance the view that the accumulation of adverse social factors (index) found in our criterion group is likely to adversely affect their speech, language and cognitive impairment. Therefore it is important to note that the correlation between this index and the children's communication code is only 0·15 and their score on the English Picture Vocabulary Test is only 0·22. However, with such low correlations we must conclude that adverse social factors appear to have less important effects than the literature has led us to expect. The correlations of the mother's language literacy index with a global measure of the child's language and a global measure of cognition are 0·11 and 0·23, which again are not impressive. Both are lower than correlations of these global measures with social class, which are 0·29 and 0·35 respectively.

3   A follow-up study: predictive importance—cognitive, language and educational development

Introduction*

The method employed in this follow-up study has been described in detail in Chapter 1. This is a study of children, with speech retardation at the age of three, who have been followed up at the age of about seven years. Material for the prospective study was gathered during a survey of the entire population of children born in 1962 in Newcastle upon Tyne (Neligan and Prudham, 1969). Speech retardation was defined as the failure to use 'three or more words strung together to make some sort of sense' (Neligan and Prudham, 1969).

This report concerns the 102 children whose parents were living in Newcastle when the children were aged three, and who were still available for study at the age of six years. As a result of the diagnostic assessment at the age of seven the study group was subdivided. One group comprised 18 children who were functionally extremely abnormal (these constituted the pathological deviant group). The remaining 84 children comprised the Residual Speech Retarded Group—the main subject of this chapter. This group of 84 children was operationally subclassified as follows (see Fig. 1):

(a) Specific Speech Delay—a group of 25 children who had speech delay but started to walk early (complete data only available on 24 cases).

(b) An intermediate group of 34 (complete data only available on 31 cases).

* A brief account of the method has been deliberately repeated in certain chapters in order to make them reasonably self-contained and thus simplify reading.

WALKING MILESTONES OF RESIDUAL
SPEECH RETARDED GROUP

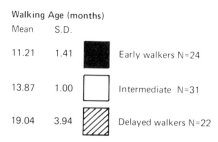

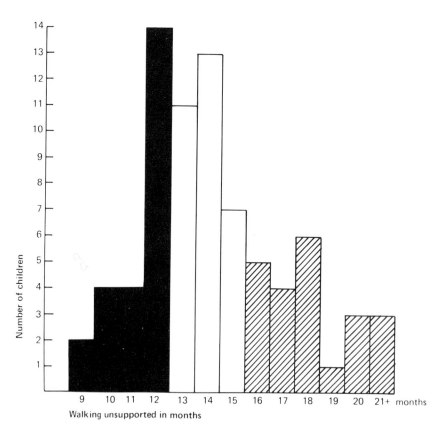

Fig. 1   Walking milestones of Residual Speech Retarded Group. In this histogram only the 77 cases with complete data were taken into account.

(c) General Milestone Delay—a group of 23 children who both walked and talked late (complete data only available on 22 cases).

As previously pointed out, the two deaf children were excluded from this classification.

The speech retarded group was matched with normal controls for age, sex and postal district.

Aim

This chapter is intended to be an account of the later development and functioning, in the three specified areas of cognition, language and education, of the 84 children who made up the Residual Speech Retarded Group. Although the main concerns of this chapter are between-group comparisons (between speech retarded and controls) some preliminary within-group comparisons are also undertaken.

It is of paramount importance to be aware of the long-term sequelae of speech retardation. There is evidence (Morley, 1965) that the use of incomplete sentences at the age of three years nine months rapidly improves, so that one year later very few children have this disability. Further, Butler et al. (1973) point out that by the age of seven years most developmental mispronunciations have disappeared spontaneously. Such apparent spontaneous improvements does not necessarily mean that henceforth all will be well, as there are reports of worrying long-term consequences. For example, the Edinburgh research group (Ingram, 1963; Mason, 1967) in their follow-up of speech retarded children in primary schools report that the majority have reading difficulties. In addition, Rutter (1972) points out that to read and 'to understand the meaning of what he reads . . . a child must have language skills'. He accordingly argues that speech delayed children are likely to have reading delays as well because both reflect language impairment. Long ago Sheridan (1948) pointed out that continuing mispronunciations betoken serious learning difficulties. Further retrospective studies of school age children with serious reading difficulties report that there is frequently a history of speech delay (Blank et al., 1968; Rutter and Yule, 1970). Such studies deal in the main with educational problems. So far, no one has attempted to ascertain systematically and comprehensively, using a prospective research technique, what are the wider consequences of speech retardation.

Method

The method has been described in Chapter 1. We have made no attempt in this study to utilize the new linguistic concepts or explore the rules of grammar and language competence (Chomsky, 1957, 1965; Menyuk, 1964, 1969; Menyuk and Looney, 1972). These measures are still clinically in their infancy and need highly specialized skills for their application. Instead, we have used traditional clinical psychological measures such as the ITPA (Kirk *et al.*, 1968) together with a wide range of measures which include tests of language expression and syntactical development. For instance, Renfrew's test (1971) was modified and scored according to criteria adapted from the work of McCarthy (1930, 1954) and Templin (1957).

In certain analyses we have excluded the two profoundly deaf children as well as two children of uncooperative families.

A brief account of the tests used and what they measure is included in Appendix 2.

Findings

Walking milestones—observed and expected findings for Residual Speech Retarded Group

On the basis of Neligan and Prudham's population survey figures (1969), the expected numbers of children who are early, intermediate or late walkers have been calculated (Table I). Comparisons reveal that very many more children than would be expected from the general population walk late. Therefore, there is a clear association between retardation of speech and walking despite excluding the pathological deviant children. Nevertheless, there are a number of children who walk early thus indicating that speech retardation is not in every case necessarily associated with a delay in learning to walk. In short, the rate of walking development of the Residual Speech Retarded Group is not

Table I   *Residual Speech Retarded Group divided according to whether the children are early, intermediate or late walkers, and analysed according to expected numbers based on the general population*

Subgroups	Observed n	Expected n	$\dfrac{(o - e)^2}{e}$
Early walkers	24	19·25	1·12
Intermediate walkers	31	50·05	7·25
Late walkers	22	7·70	26·56
Total	77	77·00	34·93

Chi-squared $= 34·93$, d.f. $= 2$, $p < 0·001$

only significantly different from that of the general population but appears to be an important criterion for differentiating between subgroups of an apparently homogeneous population of speech retarded children. Furthermore, this method of subclassifying makes it possible to effectively study the sequelae of subgroups of speech retarded children separately.

Cognitive tests

On all the cognitive (intelligence, perceptual, conceptual, visual motor) tests the Residual Speech Retarded Group had significantly poorer results than the controls (see Table 2, Appendix 1). This applied equally to the global test scores and to the subtest scores (the latter are contained in the tables in Chapter 5). The obvious interpretation is that the poorer functioning of the Residual Speech Retarded Group reflects poorer intellectual potential. In other words, both their speech delay and their poorer cognitive functioning are simply indices of wider intellectual impairment. There is the possibility that too rigorous criteria have been used to define intellectual impairment (see Chapter 1) and that the above differences are just a reflection of this. One way of checking this is by comparing the distribution of IQ scores on the WISC and ascertaining how the picture would alter by using a higher cut-off point (see Table 3, Appendix 1). It is immediately evident that the verbal and full scale IQs of the Residual Speech Retarded Group show a marked shift to the left of the distribution curve with a less pronounced shift on the performance IQ.

We had also predicted that verbal skills would be closely tied to speech delay. There was therefore the possibility that if we had used verbal intelligence as our selection criterion we would have excluded children with a reasonable intellectual and educational prognosis. The findings in Table 3, Appendix 1, appear to justify our operational decision to use the performance IQ instead. For example, it is evident that, while in the Residual Speech Retarded Group $7\frac{1}{2}\%$ of the children have verbal IQs below 70, none of the controls score as poorly as this: on the other hand, only 1% of the Residual Speech Retarded group (and none of the controls) have performance IQs below 70. Such discrepancies have great relevance in certain individual cases—for instance, one child had a verbal IQ of 69 and a performance IQ of 118 and would have been excluded from the study if the verbal IQ was the criterion. Even the use of the full scale IQ as an exclusion criterion would have been unjustified—although to a slightly lesser extent.

One explanation of the poorer functioning of the Residual Speech Retarded Group, as demonstrated in Table 3, Appendix 1, is that it is not really a homogeneous group, even though we have so far treated it as

Table II *Cognitive functioning of Residual Speech Retarded Group subdivided according to whether they walked early or late*

Measure	C = Controls (n = 100)		E = Early walkers 'specific speech' delay (n = 24)		I = Intermediate walkers (n = 31)		D = Late walkers 'general' delay (n = 22)		Significance (t test)		
	mean	s.d.	mean	s.d.	mean	s.d.	mean	s.d.	5%	1%	0·1%
Full scale IQ (WISC)	96·26	9·92	91·21	10·10	88·52	11·23	83·27	10·26	C *vs* E E *vs* D		C *vs* D C *vs* I
Performance IQ	101·17	11·04	98·96	12·87	97·74	12·91	88·64	13·29	E *vs* D I *vs* D		C *vs* I C *vs* D
Verbal IQ	92·52	9·97	85·37	9·54	84·84	9·67	81·23	7·63		C *vs* E	C *vs* I C *vs* D
Reading quotient (Schonell)	93·94	19·15	82·54	13·68	81·00	15·76	76·18	18·06		C *vs* E	C *vs* I C *vs* D
Language quotient (ITPA) (n = 101)	91·31	10·09	84·12	8·91	82·19	10·94	76·20	9·88	E *vs* D I *vs* D	C *vs* E	C *vs* I C *vs* D

such. Hence our analysis may have masked patterns specific to a subgroup. For this reason, in this chapter, we further analysed the data according to the subclassification outlined in the introduction, in terms of whether the child had a speech delay alone (specific speech delay) or a delay in both speech and walking (general delay). This constitutes a simple way of classifying the data and may not be sufficiently adequate or sensitive. Therefore in subsequent chapters we utilize other clinical and also statistical classifications.

An analysis of our findings (Table II) reveals that speech delay is a significant predictor of poor verbal and performance intelligence and of poor psycholinguistic ability and reading ability. However, this predictive power is considerably reduced for the group of children who have speech delay but walked early (their speech delay was specific). In fact, in this latter group speech delay is not predictive of performance IQ. As this group shows such a close fit on performance IQ with the controls, it can be argued that not all of the intellectual retardation which was found in the Residual Speech Retarded Group as a whole (Table 2, Appendix 1) can be explained away on the basis of a general intellectual impairment. The findings on the specific speech delayed group suggest the intellectual impairment of some children belonging to the Residual Speech Retarded Group may be specifically verbal and linguistic rather than general in nature.

For the Residual Speech Retarded Group as a whole, the WISC mean subtest profile (Fig. 2) was parallel to, but lower than, that of the controls. This appears to provide evidence of widespread impairment of abilities. Does this widespread impairment hold for the subgroups of the Residual Speech Retarded Groups—the early, intermediate and delayed walkers? It is clear that the profile of all three subgroups is, in general, depressed in relation to the controls. The profile of the early walkers is least depressed and that of the late walkers is most depressed, with that of the intermediate subgroup falling between the other two (Fig. 3).

Two main interim conclusions can be drawn: speech delay is a better predictor of impaired verbal intelligence than of performance intelligence; and combined delay in speech and walking is a good predictor of poor cognitive, language and educational development.

Later speech and language functioning

The Residual Speech Retarded Group proved to be significantly impaired on all tests of speech and language (Tables 4 and 5, Appendix 1). An analysis of these test results showed the following:

On the ITPA the Residual Speech Retarded Group showed a mean retardation of eight months compared with the controls. The profiles of both groups (Fig. 4) are roughly parallel and similar. The only points

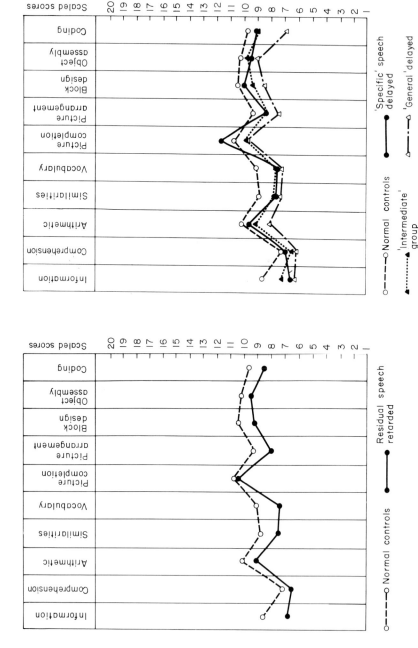

Fig. 2 (left) WISC profile of mean scaled scores for normal control and residual speech retarded groups
Fig. 3 (right) WISC profile of mean scaled scores for normal control, 'specific' speech delayed, 'intermediate' and 'general' delayed groups

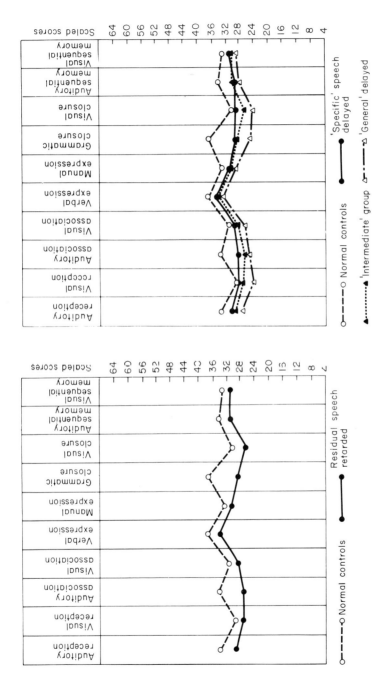

Fig. 4 (left) ITPA profile of mean scaled scores for normal control and residual speech retarded groups
Fig. 5 (right) ITPA profile of mean scaled scores for normal control, 'specific' speech delayed, 'intermediate' and 'general delayed groups'

where the profiles diverge is on Auditory Association and Grammatical Closure—where the children in the Residual Speech Retarded Group are particularly impaired. The simplest explanation of these findings is that the Speech Retarded Group show an overall immaturity of language development, but with some islands of deviant pattern of functioning as well.

Does the similarity of the ITPA profiles of the control and experimental groups also hold for the specific and general delay subgroups? Figure 5 shows that on nine of the ten subtests, each of the subgroups gave poorer results than the controls, with the general delayed (late walkers) having the worst results, the specific speech delayed (early walkers) having the best results and the intermediate group lying between these two. In addition, the.greater impairment in Auditory Association and Grammatical Closure occurs consistently in all three subgroups.

On the articulation test the Residual Speech Retarded Group as a whole not only made a greater number of errors but also used more immature speech sounds (Table 5, Appendix 1). There is therefore evidence not only of a language delay, as demonstrated by the ITPA, but also of articulatory impairment.

The communication style of the Residual Speech Retarded Group also proved to be significantly poorer; in Bernstein's (1962) terms this can be described as veering towards the restricted pole of his elaborated-restricted continuum. The salient features of Bernstein's concept of the retricted code are: an inordinate use of simple as opposed to more complex grammatical construction; poor as compared with good syntax; simple and repetitive as compared with varied and logical use of conjunctions; limited and condensed use of words as compared with varied and flexible use of words; ideas used in a stereotyped manner instead of being expressed in a flexible, clearly organized manner, and so on. Furthermore, this is the style of communication that was thought to be a consequence of poor language stimulation and associated socio-economic disadvantage (Bernstein, 1962; Deutch, 1965; Hess and Shipman, 1965; Jones and Macmillan, 1973). In our study we have already demonstrated that the social class distribution (Registrar General's) of our Residual Speech Retarded Group does not differ significantly from the controls, and we have also found that the communication style of the mothers of the children of the two groups did not significantly differ. It is, therefore, not clear why our Residual Speech Retarded Group incline towards the use of a restricted code. A plausible explanation is that there may be a number of major determinants of the restricted style of communication described by Bernstein and that speech delay in early life may be one such determinant.

Another simpler way of looking at spoken language is to assess it in terms of sentence length, completeness and complexity (Templin, 1957;

McCarthy, 1930, 1954). Here again the Residual Speech Retarded Group had poor results compared with the controls (Table 4, Appendix 1).

On the English Picture Vocabulary Test, which measures vocabulary and also provides information on the child's degree of verbal comprehension (Brimer and Dunn, 1962) the Residual Speech Retarded Group yet again had significantly poorer results than the controls.

Educational achievement

On both formal testing (Schonell Graded Word Test) and on teachers' assessments of the children's achievements at reading, writing and arithmetic, the Residual Speech Retarded Group proved to be significantly poorer than the controls (Table 2A Appendix 1). Similar findings have been reported by Ingram and Reid (1956), Ingram (1963) and Mason (1967) who followed up a group of Speech Retarded Children at school. In our study the designated subgroups again showed poorer educational achievement than the controls: results in the specific speech delayed group were better than in the intermediate group, which was again better than the general delayed group (Table II).

Imitation of gestures (Table 2, Appendix 1)

Sheridan (1969, 1972) has emphasized the importance of early imitation of activities and vocal utterances in the development of communication and the need for assessing imitative skills when assessing language functioning. Some consider (Rutter, 1972) that imitative play activities provide a 'useful guide to a child's "inner language" and basic language competence'. Such imitation and imitative play activities are usually assessed clinically only, for it requires clinical expertise to uncover such skills. The early imitation of gesture, word sounds and behaviour appears rather mechanical, but later there is a restructuring and reordering of material and increasing language comprehension. Rutter points out that, while the part played by imitation in the development of language is poorly understood and complex, serious impairment in imitation provides a warning of possible language difficulties.

There are few standardized tests with norms to assess such skills in older children (Sheridan, 1969). However, a test to measure the ability to imitate gestures of a non-symbolic nature has been devised by Berges and Lezine (1965), and a modified version of this test was used on our two groups. It was found that the Residual Speech Retarded Group was significantly poorer than the control at the imitation of gesture. This was to be expected as Rutter (1972) has pointed out that the use of gesture (imitation of gesture) is almost completely lacking in autism, only poorly present in mental retardation and moderately present in developmental language disorders. As we have already excluded children with autism and severe intellectual retardation, this finding is of considerable theoretical importance. Indeed, it is tempting to hypothesize that such poor ability to gesture may be an index of some type of receptive language disorder.

Principal component analysis of cognitive data—cognitive style (Fig. 6)

The patterns of cognitive functioning were explored further by a principal component technique. A principal component analysis was

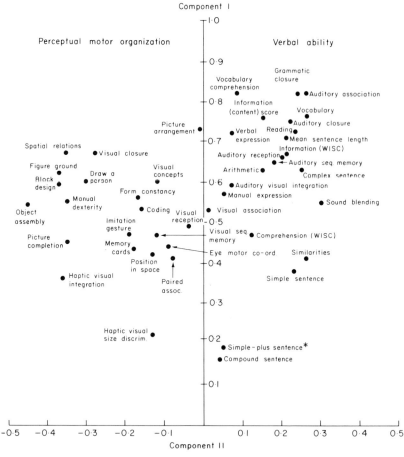

Fig. 6 Principal component analysis of cognitive data for control and residual speech retarded groups. * See p. 224 for definition.

undertaken using 44 variables from the cognitive tests (Table 7, Appendix 1). From this analysis two clinically meaningful components were derived which together accounted for 39% of the variance.

The first component was a general one and accounted for 34% of the variance. This is reasonably consistent with Vernon's (1961) conclusion that the 'g' (General) variance comprises about 40% of the variance of human abilities. It was thus conveniently labelled 'general cognitive ability'. The second component, which was bipolar, accounted for only 5% of the variance. One pole was labelled 'perceptual motor organization' and the other 'verbal ability'.

On the first component, which represents general cognitive ability, the score of the Residual Speech Retarded Group proved to be significantly lower than that of the control group (Table 8, Appendix 1). Our findings are consistent with those in other studies (Eisenson, 1971; Sheridan, 1973) with all providing evidence that, as a group, speech retarded children are lower in general intelligence than the normal population.

As was to be expected, the scores of the Residual Speech Retarded Group on the second component incline towards 'perceptual motor organization' whereas those of the controls incline in the direction of 'verbal ability' (Table 8, Appendix 1). This clearly indicates that, at the age of seven to eight, the Residual Speech Retarded Group still shows a verbal/linguistic impairment. These findings are consistent with the ITPA and WISC profiles which demonstrate that the children in the Residual Speech Retarded Group carry out non-verbal tasks relatively better than they do verbal tasks.

Allowing for environmental influences

The contribution of social environment and other associated stimulating experiences merits examination. It will be remembered that by matching for postal districts we found we had only partly controlled for social class. In Chapter 1 we described a non-significant downward gradient of social class distribution of our study groups as compared with our control group. This downward gradient is reduced when we consider the Residual Speech Retarded Group alone (by excluding that group of children with serious pathology).

We, however, considered it necessary to check that the social environmental differences between the groups was not significant and for this purpose used the more sensitive measure (described in Chapter 2) namely, the social risk index. On this measure we found significant differences between the groups which we hypothesized were determined by a clustering of adverse social factors and child handicap even within the same neighbourhood. It was therefore necessary to determine whether such an environmental risk factor made an important independent contribution to the poor performance of the Residual Speech Retarded Group. For these purposes we decided to use a partialling out technique. In brief we allocated a score of 0 to the control group and 1 to the Residual Speech Retarded Group and produced a correlation of this variable with 13 separate measures of cognitive and behavioural functioning. Of the 13 resulting correlations 11 were significant. Thereafter social risk was partialled out and we found that the correlations usually only reduce slightly but on one occasion a previously significant correlation is no longer significant and further correlation which was significant at the 0·1% level is now only significant at the 5% level. We therefore concluded for practical purposes that the social environment differences between the groups were not sufficient to substantially affect outcome. We repeated the exercise in relation to the specific speech delayed subgroup and the controls and on this occasion only found six significant correlations, which were again only very slightly affected by the partialling out technique. We therefore conclude that the social environment had virtually no independent effect in the case of this subgroup.

Discussion

Some questions remain, not all of which can be answered by our data: is the widespread cognitive and educational impairment which we found in the Residual Speech Retarded Group wholly or partially determined by the earlier speech retardation, or has some of it, at least, its basis in the same factors as those which underline speech retardation itself? Is the major part of the variance of impairment determined by adverse environmental and psychosocial factors (various types of verbal and sensory impoverishment)? Have the assessment criteria used for designating our Residual Speech Retardation Group influenced our findings? Finally, is our Residual Speech Retarded Group heterogeneous, with the influential subgroups exerting an inordinate effect on the general findings so that the lack of classification is masking the emergence of other characteristic patterns?

We have already pointed out that the ITPA profile of our Residual Speech Retarded Group is parallel but lower than that of the controls, which suggests a general impairment of language. Similar findings with the WISC profile also suggest a general cognitive impairment rather than specific impairment for the Residual Speech Retarded Group as a whole. The masking effect of lack of classification is most evident in relation to the specific speech delayed group where there is found to be a specific impairment of verbal ability. This leads on to the crucial issue of the heterogeneity of the Residual Speech Group which is discussed in detail in Chapter 5 and in other chapters on correlational analyses and multivariate techniques in the classification of speech delay.

A related question is whether the Residual Speech Retarded Group contains a subgroup of previously dysphasic children. One way of answering this question would be to take a relatively unselected cohort of children who were previously speech retarded and see if the linguistic abilities of some of them resemble that of a clinical group of dysphasic children (Olson, 1961). Although the evidence of the ITPA does not support this hypothesis, it is possible that within this Residual Speech Retarded Group there exists a subgroup of children with a dysphasic type of disorder (see Chapter 5).

As described above, social environment only makes a small independent contribution to the poor functioning of the Residual Speech Retarded Group and virtually none in the case of the specific speech delayed subgroup. While the contribution of social and other stimulation is the subject of Chapter 2, social class factors can be examined immediately. In matching for postal district we only partly controlled for social class, and thus obtained a non-significant downward gradient of social class distribution of our study group compared with our control group. However, this downward gradient is reduced even further when the pathological deviant group is excluded. A more sensitive measure of social environment was developed which we describe as the social risk index. On this index there are significant differences between our control and speech groups. We therefore considered it necessary to partial out the influence of this factor (index) and found that it had little independent effect. It is unlikely, therefore, that social class factors play any major role in the differences we have uncovered in our speech retarded group.

There are some discrepancies between our findings and the important Edinburgh follow-up of speech retarded children (Ingram and Reid, 1956; Mason, 1967). In that study the mean verbal IQ of the group was 5 points higher than the performance IQ, possibly because this was a selected group with a disproportionate number of children in the upper social classes. This leads us to speculate whether the reverse verbal–performance IQ discrepancies of that study, as compared with the current study, are an artefact of selection.

It is to be expected that in a speech retarded group there will be a number of deaf children (Morley, 1965; Greene, 1967). In fact, there proved to be two profoundly deaf children. However, not even inclusion of these two children in the audiometric analysis gave rise to statistically significant differences between the controls and the Residual Speech Retarded Group (see Chapter 5 on Audiometric Examination).

Their deafness precluded these two children from undertaking any psychological tests which included items with a verbal basis, and hence it is unlikely that hearing impairment determined any of the differences between the groups.

Conclusions

In Chapter 1 we demonstrated that one in five of a cohort of speech retarded children were seriously handicapped. If this extreme group (pathological group) is set aside, it is commonly assumed that the children in the Residual Group will soon overcome their speech disability and thereafter will function normally in most respects. However, some have shown (Ingram and Reid, 1956; Mason, 1967) that a high percentage of such children later develop educational disabilities. Our follow-up studies at the ages of seven and eight years reveal widespread cognitive, language and educational impairment including poorer intellectual ability, motor ability, imitative and intersensory skills; retarded language development; poorer articulatory ability and language skills, and a more restricted type of language expression. Principal component techniques showed that our Residual Speech Retarded Group not only had poorer 'general cognitive ability' but also inclined towards 'perceptual motor organization' whereas the controls inclined in the direction of 'verbal ability'. Such impaired functioning of children who were previously speech delayed is of major importance both diagnostically and therapeutically. It means that a child with speech delay in childhood merits careful assessment and appropriate help at school age or even earlier.

4 Predictive importance—behaviour

Introduction

The method employed in this follow-up study has been described in detail in a previous chapter. This chapter gives an account of the later behavioural development of children who, at the age of three years, were recorded as being speech retarded when compared with a matched control group (see Chapter 3).

Evidence from the literature suggests that the so-called developmental retardation syndrome may not be as benign a condition as was originally assumed. The 1000 family study (Morley, 1965) has shown that the use of incomplete sentences at the age of three years nine months rapidly improves, so that one year later very few children have this disability. Furthermore, by the age of seven years most developmental mispronunciations have disappeared spontaneously (Butler *et al.*, 1973). However, this apparent spontaneous improvement or apparent catching up does not necessarily mean that henceforth all will be well as worrying long-term consequences have been reported. The Edinburgh research group (Ingram, 1963; Mason, 1967), in their follow-up of speech retarded children when they have reached primary schools, report that the majority have reading difficulties. Rutter (1972) points out that to read and 'to understand the meaning of what he reads . . . a child must have language skills'. He accordingly argues that speech delayed children are likely to have reading delays as well because both reflect language impairment. Sheridan (1948) has commented that continuing mispronunciation indicates serious difficulties in learning. In addition, retrospective studies of school age children with serious reading difficulties frequently provide evidence of a history of speech delay (Blank *et al.*, 1968; Rutter and Yule, 1970). Such studies have mostly concerned themselves with educational sequelae, few attempting to ascertain systematically the precise behavioural consequences of, or association with, speech delay.

We already know that different facets of behaviour are highlighted by tapping different sources of information such as parents or schools (Graham and Rutter, 1970), the children themselves (Kolvin *et al.*, 1975) or direct clinical examination by a psychologist or psychiatrist. For this reason we considered it necessary to study data from all these sources.

Method

Information about behaviour and temperament, accordingly, was derived from the following sources:

(a) *Parents*—using behavioural and temperamental inventories (Kolvin *et al.*, 1975; Garside *et al.*, 1975).
(b) *Teachers*—using the Rutter 'B' Scale (1967).
(c) *Direct evidence from the child* on a self-rating personality inventory (JEPI) read out to the child by the examiner.
(d) *Direct examination by psychologist.*
(e) Systematic psychiatric examination using a modified version of the scheme proposed by Rutter and Graham (1970) simultaneously with a *physical* and *neurological* examination.

The techniques used in the above assessments are so varied that they are more conveniently described as separate introductions to each subsection.

Findings

Dimensions of behaviour and temperament (interview with parents). The parental interview questionnaires which were used to assess the behaviour and temperamental characteristics of these children are described elsewhere (Kolvin *et al.*, 1975; Garside *et al.*, 1975). As this evidence was obtained from parents, comparable ratings were available for the pathological speech retarded group.

Temperament (Table I)

Four main dimensions of temperament (Garside *et al.*, 1975) were studied—withdrawal, irregularity, mood and activity. There were no significant differences between the controls and the Residual Speech Retarded Group and the pathological speech retarded group on three of the four dimensions. The exception was the withdrawal dimension where the two speech retarded groups of children proved significantly more withdrawn than the controls (p <0·01). Further, the pathological speech retarded group proved significantly more withdrawn than the Residual Speech Retarded Group.

Dimensions of behaviour (Table I)

Here we studied four dimensions derived from factor analysis (Kolvin *et al.*, 1975), and also five additional dimensions which we considered clinically meaningful. The first four dimensions were summated to produce a global behaviour score.

   With regard to behaviour, as assessed by the parents, there were no global differences between the groups; however, the Residual Speech Retarded Group were found to be significantly different from the controls on three of the nine dimensions—they showed more motor activity (p <0·05), fewer psychosomatic symptoms (p <0·05) and poorer appetite (p <0·05). The pathological speech retarded group were found to be significantly different from the controls on four of the nine dimensions—they had more neurotic symptoms (p <0·01), fewer sleep problems (p <0·05), more bowel/bladder problems (p <0·01) and more motor activity (p <0·01). It is evident that the two study groups differ in different ways from the control group. This pattern of differences, with higher mean scores than the controls on some dimensions and lower mean scores on others, is unlikely to give rise to higher global scores. The only common pattern is the greater motor activity of the two speech retarded groups. However, it is noteworthy that, in spite of the smaller size of the sample, three of the four significant differences for the pathological speech retarded group were at the 1% level.

Items or variables of behaviour

When we studied the variables (some of which were incorporated in the dimension scores) we found that most of the differences had already emerged in the study of the dimensions and therefore few of these variables merit further description. The Residual Speech Retarded Group wet their beds, told 'lies' and pilfered significantly more frequently than the controls. The pathological speech retarded group wet and pilfered significantly more frequently than the controls (p <0·01).

   It is noteworthy that the mothers of the two speech retarded groups describe their children, at the age of seven, as having highly significant poorer enunciation than the controls. Hence, it would seem that the parents still recognize speech deficiencies in their children some three to four years after they were identified as having a speech delay.

Table I *Behaviour, temperament and personality*

Measures	a = Controls	b = Residual Speech Retarded Group	c = Pathological speech retarded group	Significance 5%	1%
A. Rutter teacher scale					
(i) antisocial	—	—	—	NS[a]	
(ii) neurotic	—	—	—	NS	
(iii) total	m 5·79	8·34	11·06		a *vs* b a *vs* c
(iv) total score 9+	24 (24%)	30 (36·1%)	9 (54%)		a *vs* b a *vs* c
9−	78	53	8		
B. JEPI					
(i) extraversion	m 18·01	16·73	NA[b]	a *vs* b	
(ii) neuroticism	—	—	NA	NS	
(iii) lie	—	—	NA	NS	
C. Temperament dimensions					
(i) withdrawal	m 16·8	19·31	22·33	b *vs* c a *vs* b	a *vs* c
(ii) irregularity	—	—	—	NS	
(iii) mood	—	—	—	NS	
(iv) activity	—	—	—	NS	
D. Behaviour dimensions					
(i) neurotic	m 13·35	13·74	16·00	NS	a *vs* c
(ii) antisocial	—	—	—	NS	
(iii) sleep	m 4·96	4·84	3·50	a *vs* c	
(iv) somatic	—	—	—	NS	
(v) bowel/bladder	m 3·44	4·00	5·08	a *vs* b	a *vs* c
(vi) motor activity	m 2·89	3·48	5·31	a *vs* b	a *vs* c
(vii) psychosomatic	m 8·24	7·44	7·73	a *vs* b	b *vs* c
(viii) phobias	—	—	—	NS	
(ix) appetite	m 3·68	3·04	3·53	a *vs* b	
total	—	—	—	NS	

For the sake of simplicity standard deviations have not been included—available on request from I.K. The data has been omitted when there are no significant differences. [a] NS = not significant [b] NA = data not available

Behaviour questionnaire completed by teachers (Table I)

The Rutter 'B' Scale has been fully described elswhere (Rutter, 1967; Rutter *et al.*, 1970a). There are three main scores—total score and two subscales—neurotic and antisocial. On evidence from the teacher, both the Residual Speech Retarded Group and the pathological speech retarded group had significantly higher (adverse) total behaviour scores than the controls (Table I). There were no differences on the neurotic or antisocial subscores.

Personality assessment (Table I)

We used the Junior Eysenck Personality Inventory (Eysenck, 1965) which has three scales—neutroticism, extraversion and lie. Again, this is extensively described elsewhere.

On this self report inventory the Residual Speech Retarded Group proved more introverted than the controls. This is in accord with the withdrawal described by the parents as reported above. (It was decided to use the method whereby the examiner read each question to the child and recorded the response so as to minimize any difficulties the child might have in reading the inventory.)

Clinical assessment by psychologist

The psychologist (Tables 9 and 10, Appendix 1) rated the children's behaviour during assessment on three three-point rating scales—attention span, level of confidence and presence of psychiatric disorder. The Residual Speech Retarded Group displayed a poorer level of confidence (p <0·01) and a poorer level of attention span (p <0·01) as compared to the controls. However, it did not prove possible to assess a sufficient percentage of the pathological deviants to make statistical analysis a valid exercise. Finally, the speech groups were rated as more psychiatrically disturbed than the controls (p <0·01) and the pathologically speech retarded group as even more disturbed than the Residual Speech Retarded Group. The rating was conducted blind as apart from the children in the pathological deviant group the membership of the remaining children was not known.

Psychiatric, physical and neurological examination

In this section we concern ourselves with direct examination of the child by a medical member of the team. The assessments comprised:

(a) A standardized psychiatric interview (Kolvin *et al.*, 1976; Wrate *et al.*, 1976; Rutter, 1967). At the end of this interview the children were rated as to whether they had 'No psychiatric disorder', 'Dubious' or 'Moderate' or 'Marked disorder'.

(b) A clinical neurological examination which is described elsewhere (Atkins *et al.* 1976) based on ratings of a series of what can be considered 'hard signs' on a three-point scale.

(c) The weight and height of the children.

Owing to shortage of resources it did not prove possible to study every child. We therefore planned a blind examination of a random sample and of approximately three-quarters of the speech retarded and control groups. The pathological speech retarded group was excluded from those examinations where it was felt it would not be appropriate or possible to carry them out in a standardized fashion. Further, the psychiatric examination of the children in the pathological speech retarded group was not conducted blind because at interviews it was usually strikingly obvious which children fell into this category as they were so qualitatively different from the others. Thus the examination of the pathological speech retarded group was of the usual clinical kind. However, the examination of the control group and the Residual Speech Retarded Group was blind—both in the sense of the interviewer not knowing from which group the child was drawn and in not having available the background information described above.

No significant differences in stature were found between the control group and the Residual Speech Retarded Group; on neurological examination the differences between the two groups were slight, although for each measure the more abnormal score was obtained by the speech group. However, our findings from the psychiatric interview clearly demonstrated a tendency for the speech group to obtain more abnormal scores on all of the measures examined; these measures include dimensions of sociability, liking of school, motor activity, *rapport* or 'accessibility' and amount of spontaneous speech. In the last three measures the differences reach statistical significance; children in the speech retarded group have less spontaneous speech at interview ($p < 0.02$), *rapport* is more difficult to establish, that is, they are more inaccessible ($p < 0.01$), and a greater number have increased motor activity ($p < 0.01$).

If the presence of mental handicap or moderate/marked mental disorder (of any type) are both included as constituting a definite psychiatric handicap then the rate of moderate or serious handicap in the total speech retarded group assessed is more than double that of the controls. These findings validate the other assessments in this section in confirming that speech delay at three has considerable predictive validity even in relation to behaviour. For the sake of economy of space, and as all cases were not assessed, it was decided not to include data tables of our findings on direct examination.

Relationship between behaviour, intelligence and language development

It has been pointed out (Lewis, 1963, 1968; Rutter, 1972) that both 'cognition' and 'socialization' have a close association with language. For instance, social anxiety and shyness are common in children with delayed or deviant language. This is particularly true, for instance, of autism and elective mutism. Further, Chess and Rosenberg (1974) report that one in four of the referrals to a psychiatric clinic had speech or language delay and of those with such delays three out of four had associated behaviour problems. Previously Leontiev and Leontiev (1959) on theoretical grounds predicted such an association, based on the fact that social interactions, which comprise one aspect of the child's behaviour, usually involve the use of language for communication and expressive purposes. A question which must then be posed is, what is the precise relationship between intelligence, language and deviant behaviour?

We studied the association between language and behaviour by correlational analysis and our findings confirm the association with a significant but not high correlation of 0.35 (p <0.01) between language and deviant behaviour (see Table 11, Appendix 1).

While it is well known that behaviour difficulties are associated with poor IQ and poor educational achievements (Yule and Rutter, 1970b) there remain crucial questions of what constitutes cause and effect. Our research was not designed to answer such questions but the fact that our Residual Speech Retarded Group's primary disorder was speech, strongly suggests that a disorder of speech and language precedes behavioural deviance. Demonstration of a high and significant relationship (Vernon, 1961, 1964) between language and intelligence in a group of children with speech and language delay supports the theory that most of the demonstrated associated deviant behaviour is secondary to cognitive and language problems. The high positive correlation which we found between the language and intelligence scores of both the Residual Speech Retarded Group ($r = 0.83, p$ <0.01) and the controls ($r = 0.74, p$ $= <0.01$), is compatible with such a theory. Moreover, both language and intelligence scores of the Residual Speech Retarded Group proved to be below average, in contrast to the average scores of the controls. However, like Mittler (1972) we are not asserting that there should always be a close relationship between language development on the one hand and intellectual development on the other. For instance, the relationship between language and intellectual development is particularly complex in certain subgroups, such as deaf children (Furth, 1971) and dysphasic children (Olson, 1961; Bartak *et al.*, 1975) and, as is shown elsewhere in this monograph, with our 'specific' speech delayed group.

Behaviour and general milestone delay and specific milestone delay

A further way of considering themes described above is by dividing the speech retarded group into those with speech delay alone (specific speech delayed group) as compared to those with delay of both speech and walking (general delayed group). On evidence from the teacher (Rutter 'B' Scale) the general delayed group displayed significantly poorer behaviour than the controls as reflected by their total scores (see Table II). While the specific speech delayed group also showed poorer behavioural adjustment, the differences were not significant. Furthermore, there were no significant differences on either the antisocial or neurotic subscales of this questionnaire.

On the Junior Eysenck Personality Inventory (a self rating questionnaire where, the tester read each question to the child so as to minimize any difficulties the child might have in reading) the intermediate and general delayed groups respectively proved significantly more introverted than the controls. Though the specific speech delayed group was also more introverted than the controls, the difference fell short of statistical significance ($p < 0.1$). There were no significant differences between the groups on the dimension of neuroticism and the lie scale.

Relationship between verbal ability and behaviour

The next question to be asked is whether poor verbal ability is associated with deviant behaviour irrespective of whether the child has a speech disorder. It was considered that a more valid answer would be obtained if we confined ourselves to a study of data from the control group. We, therefore, correlated the EPVT (English Picture Vocabulary Test) scores with 11 measures of behaviour and temperament, and found that six of these 11 measures had correlations of above 0.2 (Rutter teacher total score—0.23; irregularity of temperament—0.22; mood—0.20; neurotic dimensions—0.21; motor activity—0.20; bowel/bladder problems —0.24). Such correlations vary slightly from verbal scale to verbal scale but the highest inverse correlation was between the language quotient and the Rutler teacher total score (Table 11 Appendix 1).

Table II *Behaviour data for controls and speech retarded subgroups*

| Measures | | Groups | | | | Significance | | |
		a = Controls	b = SSD	c = IG	d = GD	5%	1%
Rutter teacher total score	m	5·8	7·3	7·3	10·2		a *vs* d
Eysenck JEPI extraversion	m	18·0	16·9	16·6	16·3	a *vs* c a *vs* d	

SSD = Specific speech delayed group; IG = Intermediate delayed group; GD = General delayed group.

Discussion

There is evidence from the literature that children with speech defects are prone to psychological difficulties. Solomon (1961) describes, on the basis of evidence from mothers, tenseness, anxiety and difficulties in interpersonal relationships. Sheridan (1973) using the Bristol Social Adjustment Guide (Stott, 1958) reports that the maladjustment rate is nearly four times that found in normal children. Rutter *et al.* (1970) approached the problem from a starting point of psychiatric disorder, and reported that boys with psychiatric disorder had double the number of speech disorders that occurred in the general population. Others assert (Rutter, 1972; Lewis, 1963, 1968) that social anxiety and shyness are common in children with language delay 'regardless of its cause' (Rutter, 1972). Ingram (1959b), in his study of children with developmental speech disorders, reported that 10 out of 80 were undergoing psychiatric treatment. He describes solitariness, withdrawal, dependency and immaturity and inappropriate reaction to frustration (tantrums or tears). Myklebust (1954) has reported similarly on children with speech disorders. However, it has been pointed out (Rutter, 1971) that the sequelae of different types of language handicaps should be studied separately and comparatively, and such studies are few (Goodstein, 1958; Lewis, 1968). Even fewer are studies of the long-term effects of earlier speech and language difficulties on behaviour. Our study provided just such an opportunity as we were able to compare groups of children with different types of speech retardation with a control group.

On the behaviour scales completed by the teachers the two groups of speech retarded children were found to be significantly more disturbed. Such disturbance bears an inverse relationship to the children's intellectual and language performance irrespective of whether the children fall into the control or the study groups. Two possible explanations spring to mind—the first is that intellectual dullness is validly related to maladjustment. Alternatively, we are witnessing the 'halo-effect' of children with comparatively poorer intellectual and language potential perceived by the teacher as showing significant excesses of disturbed behaviour.

The Residual Speech Retarded Group shows evidence of introversion and withdrawal as compared to the control group. This conclusion has support from the data derived from interview with parents in this study, the lower extraversion scores on the JEPI, poorer levels of self-confidence as perceived by the psychologist and also previous reports of withdrawal reported in the literature (Ingram, 1959a; Solomon, 1961). What we do have is evidence that multiple delays of major milestones in the earlier years of life are significantly associated with later behaviour problems. In previous chapters we have shown that the group with multiple delays have significantly poorer IQs than the controls. Hence a possible explanation for the excess of behavioural problems is that they are determined by poorer intelligence of the study groups. This suggests that the behaviour problems are, in part at least, secondary to cognitive, speech and language problems.

Summary

The weight of evidence that we have set out above provides incontrovertible proof of long-term behavioural sequelae of speech disorders in the early years of life. Those speech disorders which are more clearly pathological have by far the severest consequences. The most clear-cut pattern identified is that of speech delay and later introversion and withdrawal. When reports from teachers and the results of psychiatric assessment are considered in terms of global scores then such measures always differentiate the controls from the study groups. However, when information is obtained from parents or children then such measures do not consistently differentiate the groups.

Finally, there is evidence that severity of disturbance correlates inversely with performance on tests of intelligence and language irrespective of whether the child belongs to a study group or the control group.

5 The specific developmental speech disorder syndrome

Introduction

The specific developmental speech disorder syndrome is considered by Ingram (1972) to be a descriptive label applied to children with retardation of speech development who are otherwise normal. His views are summarized in Chapter 1. Rutter and Yule (1970) see development delays as representing 'extreme variations in normal development . . . which are related to the continuing growth and maturation of the brain'. The salient features of these delays are also noted in Chapter 1.

Ingram considers it useful for practical and theoretical purposes to regard the heterogeneous group of articulatory and language disorders that fall into this category as a spectrum of disorders which vary from the mild to the very severe. The mild disorders are the *dyslalias* which are defined as the retardation of the acquisition of word sounds but with normal language, that is, articulatory development is retarded. The moderate disorders involve normal comprehension but more severe retardation of word sound acquisition and retardation of development of spoken language, and fall into the category of *developmental expressive dysphasia*. The severe disorders involve greater degrees of retardation of word sound acquisition, impaired development of spoken language and impaired comprehension of speech, and fall into the category of *developmental receptive dysphasias* (see p. 6).

A brief review of the more recent literature on childhood dysphasia is necessary. The review by Eisenson (1968) provides a basis for an appreciation of current concepts.

Definition of childhood dysphasia

A widely accepted definition is that childhood dysphasia is a relatively specific failure of development of language and associated functions. Benton (1964), like Ingram (1972), views it as a spectrum of disorders ranging from a disability in speaking, with near normal speech and understanding, to a disability in both understanding and expression of speech. He sees the concept as one of 'specific' failure because there is no associated deafness, mental subnormality or evident neurological disability.

Clinical features

These have been variously described:

(i) *Auditory functioning* Eisenson (1966) identifies a difficulty in localization of a sound source, inconsistency of response to sounds and poorer functional hearing than would be expected from audiometric assessment. He points out that the child may have mild or moderate hearing impairment detectable by audiometry. However, such impairment is usually insufficient to account for the child's difficulty in dealing with auditory stimuli (Olson, 1961; Worster Drought, 1965) and therefore his functional hearing may be more impaired than the audiometric findings might suggest.

(ii) *Intellectual functioning* According to Eisenson (1968) the child with developmental dysphasia tends to have normal intelligence on non-verbal tests (Stark, 1967; Weiner, 1969; 1972). However, his intellectual performance tends to break down under conditions of stress or awareness of error and, in such situations, perseveration or anger reactions may supervene. Perceptual dysfunctioning occurs in one or more sensory modalities but not in all (Bartak *et al.*, 1975). Finally, the child has relatively good visuomotor functioning (Weiner, 1972).

(iii) *Speech and language functioning* Both Ingram (1972) and Eisenson (1968) suggest that dysphasic children show a spectrum of language impairment as judged by sentence length and complexity, and by grammatical or syntactical performance. Weiner (1972) reports deficiencies in repetition of vowels and sentences, and poor performance on an articulation test. In his view, these findings support the concept of difficulty in coping with the linguistic rules of grammar (Menyuk, 1964; Morehead and Ingram, 1973). Deficiencies in all aspects of auditory-vocal functioning have also been reported (Weiner, 1972).

Theoretical explanations

A wide variety of theories have been advanced to explain the problems involved in dysphasia. The contradictory nature of many of these theories often arises from the contradictions in some of the empirical evidence upon which they are based (Hardy, 1965). Such differences are brought about by many factors—for instance, the ascertainment criteria used in different studies are often different and hence the samples have not been entirely comparable or the tests used have not always been similar (Weiner, 1972).

One theory invokes the concept of defective auditory perception. The proponents of this theory contend that the main mechanism of dysphasia is a defective processing of auditory signals. Hence the dysphasic child may not be able to listen as rapidly as required to perceive and process spoken language (Eisenson, 1968).

Other theories impute both auditory perception and processing difficulties involving defects both in discrimination and in integration of auditory information. An example of this theme is that advanced by McReynolds (1966) who postulates that dysphasics have a defective capacity for storing speech sound. The essential finding is that the child is able to make correct discrimination responses for immediate but not delayed recall. Thus the child may be able to match and discriminate isolated speech sounds but not where the sound is part of a phonetic pattern. Eisenson (1968) advances a further variation on this theme consisting of a poor ability to sequence auditory events in time, and hence a defective capacity to store speech sounds (Stark, 1967; McReynolds, 1966; Monsees, 1968). Eisenson speculates that expressive dysphasia is secondary to primary receptive dysphasia. In his opinion, a child who cannot process speech has a fundamental impairment in those perceptual abilities that are essential for the understanding of language and the acquisition of speech.

Weiner (1972), on the other hand, feels there is inadequate support for Eisenson's hypothesis as the sole origin of language difficulties. He postulates instead a production difficulty which he bases on the argument that whereas normal children can imitate speech better than they can comprehend it (Fraser *et al.*, 1963), children with delayed speech comprehend grammatical structure better than they can repeat or produce it. Rees (1973) argues that the evidence for an auditory perceptual defect in language and learning disorders is limited. Instead, she proposes a cognitive deficit as the primary problem.

Another theory is that in dysphasia there is a lack of, or a delay in the development of deeper language structures (Chomsky, 1969; Lenneberg, 1966) and hence the difficulty in learning linguistic rules (Weiner, 1969). Yet another point of view is that put forward by Menyuk (1964) who attributes difficulty in coping with the rules of grammar to a deficiency in short-term memory. Perhaps this is the basis of an inability to apply principles and to generalize from one situation to another (Eisenson, 1968).

It is not surprising therefore, that there is no generally accepted theory of dysphasia. Rather, each group of workers implicates a different deficit as the central mechanism of dysphasia.

Validation of our classification of speech retardation

We have already provided a full validation of the breakdown of a group of speech retarded children into two subgroups: (1) Pathological Deviant Children; (2) Residual Speech Retarded Children. We now wish to justify our further classification of the Residual Speech Retarded (RSR) Group into subgroups comprising:

  (i) A group with specific speech delay (Specific Speech Delayed Group)
  (ii) An Intermediate Group
  (iii) A group who are delayed in both speech and walking (General Delayed Group)

Hypothesis

In this section we focus on the group with specific speech delay. This group is of great theoretical interest as not only were the children normal in all respects other than the development of speech at the age of three, but they were advanced in their walking. On theoretical grounds it seems reasonable to put forward the hypothesis that this group had suffered from *developmental dysphasia*, to at least a mild degree. We can test this hypothesis by finding to what extent their later functioning is suggestive of a developmental dysphasia according to features described in the literature. We can further test the hypothesis and validate the classification by studying the performance of the children in the three subgroups, described above in the previous section, on a number of measures and also on data available from the monitoring of these children up until the age of eight.

Findings

1 Audiometric assessment of the Residual Speech Retarded Group and the controls

When assessing children with speech and language difficulties an essential first step is to exclude deafness. Audiometry was therefore undertaken by a senior speech therapist (E.S.) using an amplivox audiometer calibrated to ISO (International Standards Organisation Zero). Each ear was tested separately. From Fig. 1 it is evident that the Residual Speech Retarded Group has slightly greater hearing loss at each frequency for the right ear with the pattern being repeated in the left ear. However, the differences are not significant and, furthermore,

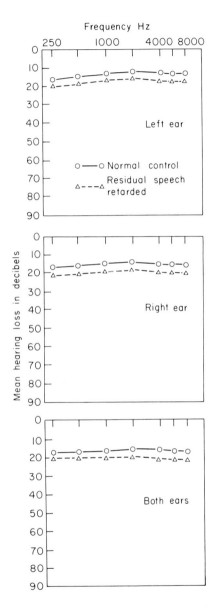

Fig. 1   Mean hearing loss in decibels at each frequency for normal control and residual speech retarded groups

the mean decibel scores fall within the normal range for each ear separately. (The data from our three separate subgroups vary only slightly from that of the Residual Speech Retarded Group as a whole and again the differences between the three subgroups and the controls are not significantly different.)

2 Global findings on cognitive testing

Table 12, Appendix 1, shows the scores achieved by the control group and three subgroups of speech retarded children on a variety of tests of cognition and language.

On all but one of the tests of cognition and on most of the tests of syntax the controls proved significantly or very significantly superior to the General Delayed Group. The only exception is on the haptic-visual integration test (of Birch) on which there is no significant difference. The controls are only significantly superior to the Specific Speech Delayed Group on four of these tests, namely, Frostig Test of Visual Perception, English Picture Vocabulary Test of comprehension, and some of the measures of syntax and language maturity—in particular information content and mean sentence length (as measured on the Bus Story Test).

The test of articulation gave some most interesting results. While the articulation of the Specific Speech Delayed Group is significantly inferior to that of the controls, that of the General Delayed Group is not.

Finally, the Specific Speech Delayed Group had better scores than the General Delayed Group on cognitive and language tests, with the exception of auditory-visual integration (Birch's Test) and haptic-visual integration (Birch's Test) and imitation of gestures. Language tests showed only one significant difference between the Specific Speech Delayed and General Delayed Groups and that was on the vocabulary comprehension test (English Picture Vocabulary Test) on which the Specific Speech Delayed Group were superior.

On a graded word reading test (Schonell) the Specific Speech Delayed Group proved to be significantly poorer than the controls but did not significantly differ from the General Delayed Group. As expected, both the General Delayed Group and the Intermediate Group were also significantly inferior to the controls.

Interim discussion

It is important to note that the Specific Speech Delayed Group, compared to the controls, do particularly well on the non-verbal tests of conceptual maturity (Draw-a-Man Test), motor ability (Purdue Peg Board), haptic-visual integration (Birch's Test), visual concepts

(Skemp's Test) and imitation of gesture . They do comparatively poorly on a test of visual perception (Frostig's Test) despite the fact that this is considered to be a non-verbal test. This is discussed later.

On the WISC of all groups the Specific Speech Delayed Group was found to have the greatest performance minus verbal IQ mean difference. The difference, which proved significantly greater than that of the control group (Table 12, Appendix 1), emphasizes the poorer verbal ability of the Specific Speech Delayed Group relative to their nonverbal ability. As expected, the Specific Speech Delayed Group also perform poorly on the test of verbal comprehension (English Picture Vocabulary Test) and their syntax is also inferior to that of the controls, though not always significantly. It was found that the Specific Speech Delayed Group used significantly more simple sentences and fewer elaborated sentences than the controls. In essence, the range of syntax and grammar of the Specific Speech Delayed Group, as expressed in their spoken language, was very much poorer than that of the control group.

Of additional importance is their inferiority to the controls on articulation, as the ages of the children at the time of this assessment was well beyond six years, which is when the majority of children in the general population are expected to have acquired normal and mature articulation (Morley, 1965; Anthony *et al.*, 1971).

Rutter (1972) points out that 'children who are delayed in talking are likely also to be delayed in reading, because both reflect language impairment'. This view is borne out by our findings for all three of our Speech Delayed Groups. Of further interest was the fact that all three Speech Delayed Groups displayed significantly greater difficulty in their ability (see Table 13, Appendix 1).:

(a) to blend units of sound (phonemes), to form words (sound blending subtest ITPA);
(b) to recognize words presented orally when one or more units of sound are omitted (auditory closure subtest ITPA).

According to D'Arcy (1973) discrimination between different units of sound forms an important aspect of learning to read. This is supported by Winitz (1966) who advances the view that 'phonemes are the elemental units of spoken language; they signal semantic distinctiveness'. Therefore, the relative poverty of the Specific Speech Delayed Group (and, indeed, of the Intermediate and General Delayed Groups) on discrimination of word sounds suggests that their reading handicap is not simply associated with poorer verbal and language ability, but also with a residual impoverishment of a more specific aspect of language, namely, word sound—or phoneme—recognition and discrimination.

The General Delayed Group was significantly inferior to the controls on almost all measures used, including verbal and non-verbal tests of cognition and on measures of language and syntax. However, the articulation of this group was not significantly inferior to that of the controls.

To sum up, the majority of the findings on the Specific Speech Delayed Group fit in with the pattern which one would expect if this group had suffered from developmental dysphasia. For example, children in this group achieved significantly better scores than those in the General Delayed Group, who are more likely to be suffering from general intellectual retardation. Further, one would have expected of the Specific Speech Delayed Group:

(i) A wide verbal–performance discrepancy on the WISC—which was found.

(ii) A near-normal level of conceptual maturity compared with the controls—which was found.

(iii) Reasonable comprehension—this would have been expected if the Specific Speech Delayed Group suffered only from an expressive dysphasic disorder with near-normal comprehension of speech. However, their significantly poorer scores on the EPVT lead to the conclusion that their disability extends beyond expression to comprehension difficulties as well.

(iv) Near-normal functioning on a test of visual perception, but this was not found. The significantly poorer performance by our Specific Speech Delayed Group as compared with the control group, on the Frostig Developmental Test of Visual Perception, raises the question of brain damage as children with varying degrees of brain damage have been reported to be inferior on this test (Maslow et al., 1964; Frostig, 1966). However, there are doubts about the validity of the Frostig as a test for brain damage and this theme is examined in some detail in Chapter 10, p. 171. We have sought corroborative evidence from clinical-neurological examination but none was found. Furthermore, there was no suggestive evidence of brain damage in our Specific Speech Delayed Group on the remaining cognitive tests.

(v) Near-normal motor functioning (on the Purdue)—which was found.

(vi) Near-normal ability to imitate (Bartak et al., 1975)—which was found.

(vii) Near-normal ability with visual concepts (on the Skemp)—which was found.

(viii) Comparatively poorer syntactical and articulatory development—which was found.

(ix) Comparatively poorer functioning on a test of education achievement—which was found.

(x) Finally, the differences between the controls and the Specific Speech Delayed Group should be narrow on performance tests, wide on verbal tests, but very much wider on tests of language and educational achievements. The actual discrepancies are according to expectation: performance IQ, 2 points; verbal IQ, 7 points; reading quotient, 12 points; language quotient, 13 points. On balance then, the weight of evidence strongly supports our hypothesis that the children in the Specific Speech Delayed Group have a pattern of cognitive functioning reminiscent of a continuing developmental dysphasic disorder. On the other hand, the pattern of the General Delayed Group is that of widespread cognitive impairment, syntactical impairment but not articulatory impairment. This strongly supports the view that this group is suffering from general retardation rather than a more circumscribed impairment.

3 Cognitive tests—pattern of subtest scores

(a) ITPA subtests

The next step was to study the psycholinguistic abilities of the three subgroups on the assumption they would show differences in profile and patterns of subtest scores which might provide clues to the nature of the language deficit in the three subgroups. Figure 2, which compares the profiles of the subtests of the ITPA, reveals that compared to the control group:

(i) The General Delayed Group have significantly poorer results on each of the ten subtests. This is similar for the Intermediate Group, except on the subtest measuring visual reception on which they did not significantly differ from the controls (Table 13, Appendix 1).

(ii) The Specific Speech Delayed Group have significantly poorer results than the controls on four subtests—auditory association, verbal expression, grammatic closure and auditory sequential memory. They do not differ from the controls on those tests which rely heavily on the interpretation of tasks involving the visual modality, but differ significantly on those that rely on the auditory modality. The one exception to this pattern is the auditory reception subtest where the differences between the controls and the Specific Speech Delayed Group approach the 5% level of significance only. Furthermore, the Specific Speech Delayed Group was not significantly superior to the Intermediate Group on any subtest.

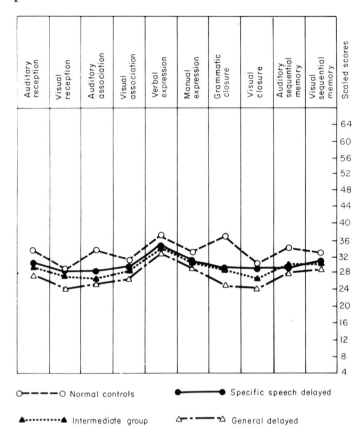

Fig. 2 ITPA profile of mean scaled scores for normal control, 'specific speech delayed, intermediate and general delayed groups

Interim discussion

At the age of seven, the three subgroups of speech retarded children have residual linguistic difficulties. The extent of the difficulties is closely tied to their previous prowess or delay in walking.

The Specific Speech Delayed Group are significantly inferior to the controls on tasks which are heavily reliant on auditory or verbal functioning, but not on tests which are dependent on visual input (visual reception, visual association, visual closure, visual sequential memory) or on motor or manual language output (manual expression). It is of importance to note the tests in which these children have residual specific difficulties. These include:

    (i) description of familiar objects—e.g. ball, an envelope, etc. (verbal expression);

 (ii) correct completion of a statement in which grammatical elements such as plurals, tenses, comparatives and superlatives are the key features (grammatical closure);

 (iii) completion of a verbal statement according to an understanding of verbal analogies, e.g. 'bread is to eat, milk is to . . .?' (auditory association);

 (iv) production from immediate memory of sequences of digits (auditory sequential memory). Children in the Specific Speech Delayed Group therefore have poorer language abilities than would be expected from their global intelligence.

The poor performance on grammatic closure is in accord with the view that dysphasics have difficulty in coping with the linguistic rules of grammar (Menyuk, 1964; Lenneberg, 1966). The inferior performance on tests which heavily rely on the auditory modality is consonant with the contention that dysphasic children have a basic defect in processing and sequencing auditory signals, that is, that they suffer from a form of auditory imperception (Eisenson, 1968; Stark, 1967). In this respect, it is interesting to note that the Specific Speech Delayed Group did badly on the test of auditory sequential memory but not on the test of visual sequential memory.

  In summary, the overall pattern of tests on the ITPA again supports the hypothesis that the Specific Speech Delayed Group previously suffered from a type of developmental dysphasia.

(b) WISC subtests

Our results are presented in both tabular (Table 14, Appendix 1) and graphical form (Fig. 3). The pattern of WISC subtest scores from the various groups are broadly similar. The main findings are:

 (a) The General Delayed Group is significantly inferior to the controls on eight of the ten subtests and the difference on another subtest, object assembly, just falls short of statistical significance.

 (b) The Intermediate Group is significantly poorer than the controls on six subtests, four of which belong to the verbal scale.

 (c) The Specific Speech Delayed Group is significantly poorer than the controls on four subtests, three of which are verbal (information, similarities and vocabulary) and on one performance subtest (picture arrangement).

 (d) The General Delayed Group is significantly poorer than the Specific Speech Delayed Group on arithmetic (verbal scale) and on picture completion, block design and coding (performance scale). Thus the Specific Speech Delayed and General Delayed

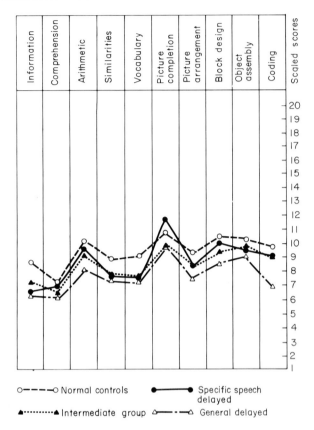

Fig. 3 WISC profile of mean scaled scores for normal control, specific speech delayed, intermediate and general delayed groups

Groups are differentiated from each other mainly by their differing abilities to carry out non-verbal tasks.

Intellectual functioning and 'dysphasia'

There are comparatively few reported studies on the *specific* intellectual abilities and impairments of dysphasic children. In this section our aim, therefore, is to compare patterns of impairment as displayed by our Specific Speech Delayed Group with the clinical descriptions of dysphasic children as described in the literature. The pattern of intellectual functioning of our Specific Speech Delayed Group is based on their performance on the WISC. This battery consists of 12 subtests, 10 of which have been used in our study, and thus allows for a pattern approach (Cohen, 1959; Glasser and Zimmerman, 1967; Sattler, 1974).

As a basis for interpreting our WISC findings we have decided to use Cohen's Factor Analytical Model, with particular reference to the analysis at $7\frac{1}{2}$ years which is the age which is most relevant to our study. The major factors defined by Cohen (1959) are shown in Table I. Cohen sees *verbal comprehension I factor* as a reflection of verbal knowledge influenced mainly by 'formal education', and *verbal comprehension II* as 'the application of judgement to situations following some implicit verbal manipulation'. The *perceptual organization factor* is regarded as a non-verbal factor which reflects the ability to interpret and/or organize visually perceived material against time and the *freedom from distractability factor* as a measure of the ability to attend or concentrate.

Table I *Subtest with loadings of important primary factors* (derived from Cohen, 1959)

	Factor A	Factor B	Factor C	Factor D
Subtest	information	picture arrangement	arithmetic	comprehension
	arithmetic similarities	block design object assembly	digit span[a] picture arrangement	vocabulary picture completion
	vocabulary	mazes[a]		
Interpretation	verbal comprehension I	perceptual organization	freedom from distractability	verbal comprehension II

[a] We did not include these subtests in our study

Using the interpretation proposed by Cohen (1959) we can attempt to describe the nature of intellectual functioning of our Specific Speech Delayed Group as highlighted by their score on each of the WISC subtests. We have used a simple method which involved grouping the subtests under the factor headings proposed by Cohen. We have then compared the scores of the Specific Speech Delayed Group and control group on the subtests in terms of their particular factor grouping. Our findings show that on all four subtests which constitute the *verbal comprehension I factor* as described by Cohen, our Specific Speech Delayed Group do poorly, significantly so on three of them (that is, on information, similarities and vocabulary). As for Cohen's *verbal com-*

prehension II factor, our Specific Speech Delayed Group again do worse than the controls, though significantly so on only one of the three subtests (that is, on vocabulary) with important loadings on this factor.

The only subtest of the WISC non-verbal scale on which our Specific Speech Delayed Group are significantly poorer than the controls is picture arrangement. Further, it is of interest to note that this subtest forms both part of Cohen's *perceptual organization factor* and of the *freedom from distractability factor* at the age level of $7\frac{1}{2}$ years.

In summary, then, the specific area of intellectual impairment of our Specific Speech Delayed Group is predominantly in the sphere of verbal reasoning in terms of both verbal comprehension factors described by Cohen. This is in general agreement with clinical and other findings in studies of dysphasic children (Eisenson, 1968; Weiner, 1972; Bartak *et al.*, 1975). To a lesser extent there are deficits of perceptual organization and concentration as measured by the picture arrangement subtest. We accept that the latter interpretation is based on the strength of only one subtest and it therefore must be viewed with caution. Nevertheless, this finding is reminiscent of Eisenson's (1968) observation that dysphasic children are inclined to lose sight of the principle necessary for completion of a task which in our view constitutes a form of distractability.

Rank order and gaps between WISC subtests

Another way of studying our data is to compare the rankings of the mean subtest scores of the groups studied. The rankings are shown in Table II. It will be seen that, on the verbal scale, rankings of the Intermediate Delayed Group and the General Delayed Group are similar to those of the controls. Interestingly, our Specific Speech Delayed Group and Rutter's dysphasic group have identical rankings. However, on the performance scale it is our Specific Speech Delayed Group and the controls that have identical rankings while the General Delayed Group and Rutter's dysphasic group have similar but not identical rankings.

After ranking the mean subtest scores and using the studentized range statistic (Q) for correlated data and testing for a significant gap between subtests we found that:

(a) On the WISC verbal subtests the gap between arithmetic and comprehension for the controls was significant ($p < 0.01$). For the Specific Speech Delayed Group there was a significant gap between arithmetic on the one hand, and information, comprehension, vocabulary (all $p < 0.01$) and similarities ($p < 0.05$) on the other. For the General Delayed Group the only significant gap

Table II   *Ranked order of mean scores on subtests of WISC*

	Controls	SSD	ID	GD	Rutter's dysphasics
Verbal					
Arithmetic	1	1	1	1	1
Vocabulary	2	3	2	3	3
Similarities	3	2	3	2	2
Information	4	5	4	4	5
Comprehension	5	4	5	5	4
Performance					
Picture completion	1	1	1	1	2
Block design	2	2	3	3	1
Object assembly	3	3	2	2	3
Coding	4	4	4	5	5
Picture arrangement	5	5	5	4	4

SSD = Specific Speech Delayed Group; ID = Intermediate Delayed Group; GD = General Delayed Group.
High rankings e.g. 1,2,3 = higher mean scores; low rankings e.g. 8,9,10 = lower mean scores

was between arithmetic and comprehension ($p < 0.05$). These findings simply suggest that the Specific Speech Delayed Group have a specific verbal deficit.

(b) On the WISC performance subtests for the controls there was no significant gap between the tests. For the Specific Speech Delayed Group the mean for picture completion was significantly higher than that for picture arrangement ($p < 0.01$). For the General Delayed Group the mean for picture completion was again significantly higher than that for picture arrangement ($p < 0.05$) and for coding ($p < 0.01$). This suggests that these two latter groups have an impairment on Cohen's factors B, C or both.

In summary, the pattern of verbal scale subtests of the WISC suggests that the Specific Speech Delayed Group and control group were performing differently. Some workers (Eisenson, 1968) have suggested that the dysphasic child performs patchily on intelligence tests. Looking at the graphs of subtests both on the WISC and the ITPA it is evident that the profiles of the speech groups are very similar to that of the controls but more depressed. A suggestion of pacthiness, though not marked, is evident in our Specific Speech Delayed Group. However, there are degrees of dysphasia and it is only the extreme cases that are likely to show most of the characteristics described in the literature (Oslon, 1961; de Ajuriaguerra, 1966; Eisenson, 1968; Weiner, 1972; Bartak *et al.*, 1975). As it is unlikely that our Specific Speech Delayed Group have a severe degree of dysphasia they cannot be expected to show all the features described but at least they show verbal impairment and possibly distractability.

Rank order and gaps between ITPA subtests

The exercise described above can be repeated in relation to the ITPA subtests (Table III). The differences in patterns of rankings are immediately evident. First, on the auditory association subtest the three speech groups have low rankings (in other words, have low scores) compared to those of the controls; second, on the grammatic closure subtest the three speech groups rank low compared to ranking of the controls; and, third, on the manual expression subtest, the three speech groups rank high whereas the controls rank low. These findings suggest that all three speech groups do badly on auditory sequential memory, auditory association and also on grammatic closure, but that they do relatively well on manual expression. Table III, therefore, highlights the findings reported in Chapter 3.

Table III *Ranked order of mean scores on subtests of the ITPA*

	Controls	SSD	IG	GD
Verbal expression	1	1	1	1
Grammatic closure	2	7	6	7
Auditory sequential memory	3	5	4	4
Visual sequential memory	4	2	2	3
Auditory association	5	10	10	8
Auditory reception	6	4	5	5
Manual expression	7	3	3	2
Visual association	8	6	7	6
Visual closure	9	8	9	10
Visual reception	10	9	8	9

See footnote to Table II

When we tested for a significant gap between pairs of subtests within each of the groups, as described previously, we found:

(a) *Controls* The mean scores of verbal expression and grammatic closure are both significantly higher than those of manual expression (p <0·05), visual association (p <0·05) and visual closure and visual reception (p <0·01).

(b) *Specific Speech Delayed Group* The mean score on verbal expression is significantly higher than the lowest mean scores on six of the remaining subtests. The high ranking on the verbal expression subtest may seem surprising. However, as this is mainly a test of ability to name and describe the salient features of common place objects (e.g. button, envelope) rather than a test of wide-ranging verbal expressive fluency, we do not consider that very much importance ; hould be attached to this subtest.

(c) *General Delayed Group* The pattern is roughly similar to that of the Specific Speech Delayed Group in terms of a significant gap between the mean score verbal expression (which is ranked highest) and the lowest mean scores on six of the remaining subtests. While this technique is intended to identify the pattern of subtest scores *within each group* and not to compare mean subtest scores between groups, the findings on this subtest are of little importance for the reasons given above.

Conclusion

We have demonstrated that, among the wider population of children who suffer from speech delay at the age of three years, there is a subgroup of children who have no demonstrable neurological disorder, who are of normal non-verbal intelligence and whose differences from the controls cannot be attributed to an adverse social environment, as this had been controlled.

Hence this group, with specific speech delay, can be considered to be suffering from a continuing developmental speech disorder and can credibly be categorized as a specific developmental dysphasic group. Such children have not only articulation problems but also a number of other significant impairments. The pattern of impairments is not clear-cut—and this is evident from those subtests which require varying degrees of comprehension for their successful completion. On the one hand there are significant deficits on relevant subtests of the Illinois Test of Psycholinguistic Abilities (such as auditory association, grammatic closure and auditory sequential memory), of the WISC (information, vocabulary and similarities) and on the English Picture Vocabulary Test. On the other hand, there are important subtests on which no significant impairments occur and these include the ITPA (such as auditory reception, visual association and visual closure) and the WISC (comprehension).

In addition, the Specific Speech Delayed Group, compared with the controls, displays inconsistent expressive language deficits—for instance, on the ITPA they have a significant deficit of verbal expression but no impairment of manual (motor) expression. Thus the language disabilities of the Specific Speech Delayed Group are of a mixed variety—they include defects in comprehension and expression of language. Such defects are patchy but nevertheless appear mainly to occur in relation to the auditory and vocal modalities as opposed to the visual and motor modalities.

Some workers have demonstrated that dysphasics have difficulty in ordering or sequencing material. Children in our Specific Speech Delayed Group have difficulties in relation to auditorily presented material. There is no evidence of motor difficulty (on the Purdue Pegboard) and little evidence of visuo-spatial difficulty. Bartak et al. (1975) found articulation deficits in their dysphasic group and we have found similar deficits in our Specific Speech Delayed Group. On the other hand, our General Delayed Group has proved to be delayed or impaired on almost all tests used but did not have significant defects of articulation.

It would seem that there are at least two clearly identifiable sub-groups: first, those who start with specific delay and end with a pattern of functioning reminiscent of the syndrome of developmental dysphasia described in the literature; second, those who are delayed both in speech and walking and who are subsequently found to function poorly on nearly all the tests used except that of articulation.

The above findings amply demonstrate that outcome is closely tied to the generality of impairment as indicated by delay on development milestones.

In a previous chapter we report that a quarter of the speech retarded children had had specific speech delay. We therefore calculate that specific speech delay occurs in 1% of the child population.

In some ways our findings are unsupported by the work of others. For instance, Lenneberg et al. (1964) studied children with Down's syndrome, and found a strong relationship between language development and motor development especially with regard to age of walking and this is reminiscent of our General Delayed Group. On the other hand, as Mittler (1972) points out, late language development does not necessarily imply subnormality of intelligence. Our research helps to clarify the picture by distinguishing between groups of children—one with specific delay of speech who have greater potential for catching up, and the other with delay in both speech and walking who later prove to have widespread impairment.

6 Correlational and cluster analysis

Aim

The main aim of this chapter is to take a preliminary look at the inter-correlations of some of the fundamental data on our group of Residual Speech Retarded Children. This can be done by studying significant inter-correlations within the correlation matrix and also by a simple cluster analysis of variables.

Method

Thirteen variables in all were used and the rationale for their choice is described in the next chapter. The variables can be roughly grouped as follows:

(a) *Social factors and sex*
  1 Social class
  2 Language literacy index of mother as rated by social interviewer
  3 Sex of child
(b) *Physical and developmental factors*
  4 Right–left differentiation difficulties as rated by psychologist
  5 Hearing impairment as rated audiologically
  6 Test of audiovisual integration (Birch and Belmont, 1964; Kahn and Birch, 1968)
  7 General milestone delay
(c) *Cognitive and language factors*
  8 English Picture Vocabulary Test (EPVT)
  9 Usage of communication code by the child (cf. Bernstein, 1962)
  10 Test of Ability to Imitate Gestures (Berges and Lezine, 1965)
  11 Ratings of number of immature errors of articulation
  12 WISC scatter score (as defined on p. 157)
  13 ITPA scatter score

Cluster analysis

One way to identify associations between variables is to use cluster analysis of these variables. The method used on this occasion was the Elementary Linkage Analysis of McQuitty (1957) which was described by Philip and McCulloch (1966) as a rapid and objective method for clustering variables into types. It is dependent on the highest level of association which any one variable has with any of the other variables. Following Kolvin *et al.* (1973a) modifications were adopted as follows:

- (i) All correlations below 0·24 were excluded (p <0·02 approximately).
- (ii) Variables with the highest inter-correlations were used to label the cluster.
- (iii) All the rest of the modifications described elsewhere (Kolvin *et al.*, 1973a) proved irrelevant on this occasion. However, all the previously outlined cautions about this type of analysis remain valid.
- (iv) Variables from the correlation matrix of Table 15, Appendix 1, were used, but for cluster analysis purposes the variables have been recoded so that a high score indicates a positive quality (see next chapter).

The main cluster identified has been labelled a cognitive cluster (Fig. 1) with a specific focus on vocabulary comprehension as reflected by the English Picture Vocabulary Test. Indeed, the cluster demonstrates the signal importance of comprehension impairments in our Residual Speech Retarded Group. The internal associations within the cluster are clinically meaningful and plausible theories can usually be offered to explain them.

The three main cognitive measures deliberately selected for this analysis consisted of vocabulary comprehension, auditory visual integration and communication code which tap processes basic to language function. Hence, it is not surprising that these constitute a triad with the highest inter-correlations (Fig. 1). However, the salient feature of this analysis is the central and pivotal nature of the measure of vocabulary comprehension which correlates significantly (though not highly) with the majority of the remaining variables. The internal associations within this cluster merit theoretical explanation. The overall importance of *vocabulary comprehension* may be due to it being the central feature of a dysphasic syndrome in a subgroup of children within the Residual Speech Retarded Group; its associations are: gender in terms of a higher proportion of boys to girls; less in the way of hearing impairments; better occupational social class distribution of the family; greater scatter on the WISC subtests (which has been described in childhood dysphasia by de Ajuriaguerra, 1966) and, finally, relatively good motor milestone

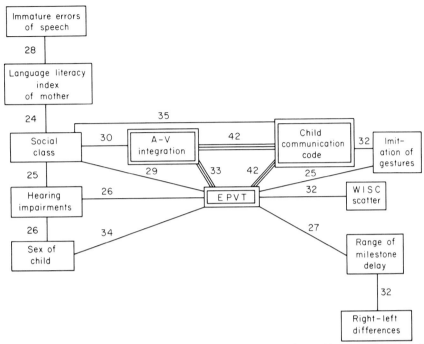

Fig. 1 Cognitive cluster (focuses on comprehension). A–V = audio visual integration; EPVT = English Picture Vocabulary Test. All measures have been scored in the same direction. Treble lines indicate the key links; variables with double margins are key chosen variables. Only significant correlations are included. Immature errors of speech, Hearing impairments, Right–left differences are positive scores (i.e. 'absence of').

development.

The sub-cluster which includes the variable 'language literacy index of mother' merits particular comment. It is discussed further in the next chapter but the feature of particular note is the association between poor language literacy index of the mother and the immature errors of articulation in the child. Does this mean that immature errors are related to slow or uneven developments of speech and language or are they at least in part artefacts of inadequate speech 'training' or conditioning by mothers from poor environments? We would like to hypothesize from these findings that the influence of a poor environment cannot be ignored but our method does not permit firm statements about causal relationships.

Discussion of correlational analysis (see Table 15, Appendix 1)*

Comment will only be made on those associations which were not discussed in the section on cluster analysis.

* Note that the variables have not been recoded in this table.

It will be seen that social class correlates significantly but not highly with the language literacy index of the mother (0·24) and the child's communication code (0·35). From the literature (Bernstein, 1962; Hess and Shipman, 1965; Jones and McMillan, 1973) one would have expected much higher correlations between social class and these other features. Furthermore, the language literacy index of the mother bears no relationship here to the child's communication code. This is surprising, especially as the principles employed in developing both measures were broadly similar. On the other hand, the language literacy index of the mother correlates positively with the articulatory ability of the child and with the child's achievements on the auditory visual integration test. Social class correlates with the test of comprehension (the EPVT) and also with intersensory integration as measured by the auditory visual test. These findings can be interpreted in a number of ways. First, our language literacy score may not be an adequately sensitive measure of mother's language literacy skills. Alternatively, it may be that widespread influences of social factors make a greater contribution to the child's cognitive development than do mother's language literacy characteristics alone.

Over 25% of the other inter-correlations are statistically significant and some merit special comment. While scatter on the ITPA has no significant correlations, scatter on the WISC correlated with the EPVT and auditory visual integration. Why do higher scatter scores go with higher achievements on the two measures of cognition that we have included? One explanation is that if the children scored evenly on the WISC they would obtain a low scatter score; if they did patchily better on certain subtests they would obtain a high scatter score; hence a high scatter score may represent considerable unevenness of abilities. This may occur with children of either good or poor intellectual potential provided they have some special skills. It can also be argued from previous research that such unevenness of abilities is likely to occur in that group of children with dysphasic difficulties (Olson, 1961; de Ajuriaguerra, 1966). If this latter explanation has any validity then a number or a subgroup of children in the Residual Speech Retarded Group must be viewed as having residual speech and language difficulties of a dysphasic nature.

A contribution to our understanding of the associations of our measure of comprehension within the Residual Speech Retarded Group can be gleaned from checking correlations with the non-cognitive variables used in other analyses. The EPVT in fact correlates significantly with a family history of development difficulties (–0·30).

The above correlations are consistent with a dysphasic syndrome in a subgroup of children within the Residual Speech Retarded Group. Some of the previously described clinical features of such a syndrome are reminiscent of the correlations described above and include the male preponderance, a high family incidence of developmental difficulties, evidence of milestone delay, right/left orientation difficulties, comprehension difficulties and an association with a fairly wide scatter on the WISC.

7 Multivariate techniques and classification of speech delay

Introduction

This chapter, in many ways, summarizes complex arguments previously mentioned and therefore, in order to make it clear for our readers, we shall repeat the salient features of the method. The total population of children born in Newcastle upon Tyne in 1962 were screened to identify those who proved to be speech retarded at the age of three years (as reported by health visitors). The speech retarded group comprised 102 children who were studied at six years and again at seven years and the control group comprised 102 children still living in Newcastle at the age of seven. They had been matched for age, sex and neighbourhood (postal district). Of the 102 speech retarded children a subgroup was identified whose functioning was so abnormal that they had to be analysed separately. This latter group constitutes what we have labelled the pathologically deviant group and the remaining children have been labelled the 'Residual Speech Retarded Group' or, alternatively, the 'developmental speech disorder syndrome group'. Unlike Ingram (1972) we made no specification about intelligence or home background in our definition of the developmental speech disorder syndrome.

Aim of the present chapter

It is commonly assumed that speech delayed children constitute a homogeneous group, the majority of whom improve spontaneously by the time they go to school, but a small remainder will suffer from the consequences of this early delay. However, this has now been disproved by other workers (Ingram, 1963; Mason, 1967; Morley, 1965; Rutter 1967) and by our own research. It is clear, in fact, that children who have speech delay at three are a heterogeneous group (Ingram, 1972). The aim of this chapter is to attempt to delineate relatively separate subgroups within this Residual Speech Retarded Group.

This is a particularly difficult exercise because, although this is a longitudinal study, there were long gaps when the children were not under scrutiny so that it can more accurately be described as a series of cross-sectional assessments. While one systematically gathers evidence at these cross-sectional assessments there are times during which unmonitored major changes may take place. In these circumstances assessment is tied to current available data and can only cautiously draw on retrospective data.

Method

Two major approaches have been used in the past to classify behaviour. First, there is the time-honoured but not necessarily scientifically validated clinical approach. Second, there is the multivariate approach pioneered in relation to child psychiatric disorders by Hewitt and Jenkins (1944) and subsequently extensively used (Kolvin *et al.*, 1973a; Garside *et al.*, 1975).

Clinical approach to classification

Here the clinician carefully sifts the data associated with the child's early life experiences, social background features, other biological phenomena and natural history and then comes to a clinical decision about identifiable subdivisions. He can then in a particular series ascertain if the features of the subgroups that he has identified statistically hang together by means of simple quantitative or qualitative comparisons.

The central question is whether speech retarded children are a homogeneous group. First, we had isolated the pathological deviant group comprising children whose functioning was so abnormal that it had to be analysed separately. Even this group is not internally homogeneous from the clinical point of view (see previous chapter). This leaves the Residual Speech Retarded Group which we consider has many characteristics in common with the developmental speech disorder syndrome as described by Ingram, provided we ignore his stipulation that the children have to be of 'average or above average intelligence' and must come from normal home backgrounds. We further consider that this group may comprise a number of clinical subgroups such as: a subgroup with general milestone delay (i.e. delay in speech and walking) and a subgroup with specific milestone delay (i.e. delay in speech alone).

At this stage we had no way of ascertaining whether these two subgroups were mutually exclusive or overlapping, and whether there were features which were characteristic of these subgroups. If the latter were the case, it might well be that we could identify a number of relatively discrete syndromes. There is no ideal way of solving the problem which presented at this stage. The solution which we devised was two-fold. First, to identify the children falling into the two subgroups described above and then to find out the extent of the differences between the subgroups themselves and between each subgroup and the remaining group of children.

Factor analytical approach

After allocation of children to one of these two subgroups, discriminant function analysis was undertaken in an attempt to pinpoint the features which discriminate the subgroups from each other. A further statistical solution consists of analysis of selected features in order to ascertain whether statistically determined factors can be identified which are clinically meaningful. The most common statistical technique for such purposes is factor analysis which clusters features rather than people, and for theoretical reasons we have preferred to use the method of principal component analysis.

In the following sections, after the preliminary correlation analysis, we have recoded all variables so that a high score always indicated a positive value in the sense of good social and family functioning or achievements on psychological or other tests. For the sake of simplicity we have presented only selections of the multivariate analysis data, in table or graph form.

Ingram, one of the leading authorities on the subject of classification of speech and language disorders in childhood, hoped that such classification would eventually be primarily based on linguistic and phonetic criteria (Ingram 1972). Until this could be achieved he considered it practical (and expedient) to base his classification on the disordered speech function and associated clinical findings. We doubt if what is in essence a unifactorial classification (i.e. based on linguistic and phonetic criteria alone), without consideration of associated clinical phenomena, would have sufficient compass to do justice to Ingram's secondary speech disorders category. Nor would such a typology have adequate aetiological, or possibly even therapeutic, utility. In brief, whatever the linguistic and phonetic basis of a typology, it undoubtedly

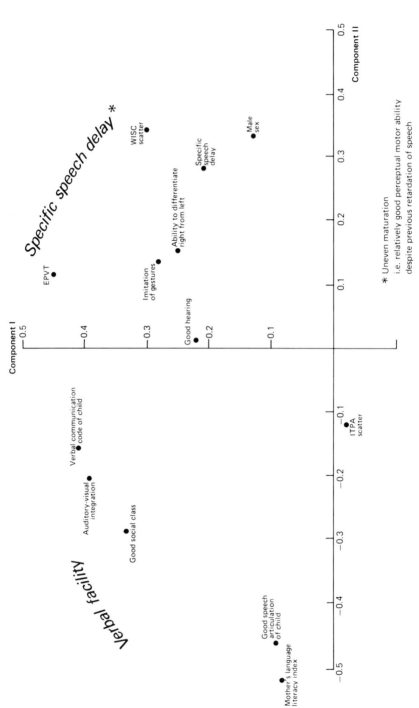

Fig. 1 First principal component analysis (Residual Speech Retarded Group)

must take into account associated clinical and environmental phenomena.

In the multivariate analyses we adopted a multiple stage strategy. The first stage consisted of utilizing the 11 key measures delineated below. To these we added social class and sex to make up 13 variables in all. The variables can be arbitrarily grouped as follows:

(a) *Social factors*
  1 Social class
  2 Language literacy index of mother as rated by social interviewer
(b) *Physical cum developmental factors*
  3 Sex
  4 Right–left differentiation difficulties as rated by psychologist
  5 Hearing impairment as rated audiologically
  6 Milestone delay (ranging from specific speech to general delay)
(c) *Cognitive cum language factors*
  7 English Picture Vocabulary Test (EPVT)
  8 Usage of communication code by the child (cf. Bernstein, 1962)
  9 Test of Ability to Imitate Gestures (Berges and Lezine, 1965)
  10 Ratings of frequency of immature errors of articulation
  11 WISC scatter score (as defined on p. 157)
  12 ITPA scatter score
  13 Audiovisual integration (Birch and Belmont, 1964; Kahn and Birch, 1968)

Principal component analyses

First principal component analysis—Residual Speech Retarded Group only (Table 16, Appendix 1, and Fig. 1)

This included only those 71 cases in the Residual Speech Retarded Group that had full data on every one of the 13 variables. As we had a relatively small sample we decided to concentrate on the first two components only.

The first component is a general one of social factors and cognitive achievements and takes up 21% of the variance. The second component is bipolar and takes up 13% of the variance; we have interpreted it as a pole of verbal facility and social influences versus a pole of uneven maturation (i.e. specific speech delay). The former is represented by the mother's language, the child's communication code, good speech and articulation and parental social class; and the latter represented by a specific delay of speech (as opposed to general delay of milestones), ability to differentiate between right and left side of the body, to imitate gestures, a high WISC scatter score and, finally, sex of child (boys). In other words, this pole is represented by relatively good motor perceptual abilities but poor verbal abilities. All these features could be considered to be a cluster representative of uneven maturation which has been described as occurring in greater or lesser degrees in groups of children clinically diagnosed as dysphasic.

Second principal component analysis—Residual Speech Retarded Group only (see Table 17, Appendix 1)

The second set of variables used for principal component analysis were 22 in number. These included a series of cognitive variables, social class, mother's language literacy index, a series of measures of social functioning, milestone delay, hearing, right–left differentiation abilities and good speech and articulation of the child. The first two components took up some 46% of the variance. As in the previous analysis, the first component is a general one with the high loadings occurring almost entirely on the cognitive variables. The second component is bipolar. At one pole are features representative of language literacy of mother, a number of measures of the child's syntax (e.g. sentence complexity) and verbal communication code and also social factors. At the other pole are a combination of measures of non-verbal abilities such as WISC performance IQ, visual concepts or visual perception, right–left differentiation ability, together with specific speech delay (Fig. 2).

Interim comment

In both principal component analyses, but especially in the first, where a lesser number of variables are used, the general factor represents positive environmental experience, early development and high achievements which all vary together. But we also have clear factorial evidence, on the second component, of a clustering of features representative of uneven maturation, i.e. specific speech delay. These are all meaningful findings and will be discussed in detail later.

Third principal component analysis—Residual Speech Retarded Group only

The next set of variables included the original 13 plus another 11 of behaviour as tested or perceived by teachers (Rutter), parents (behaviour and temperament) and the child (JEPI). The first component

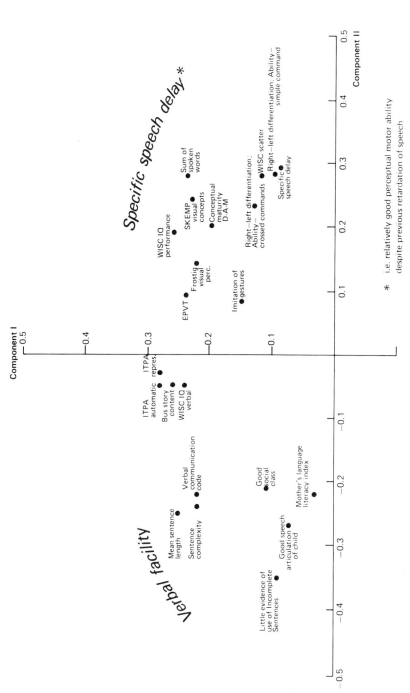

Fig. 2   Second principal component analysis

extracted was again a general one with the highest loadings on cognitive and behavioural variables taking up 16·3% of the variance. The second was bipolar taking up 11·3% of the variance. At one pole the highest loadings were of language and other cognitive and behavioural variables and at the other pole were features again representative of uneven maturation. As this analysis is similar to that for other components, we have not described it in detail or provided a table.

Final overall principal component analysis

From the previous principal component analyses we selected 33 variables for a final overall principal component analysis, combining cases falling into the Residual Speech Retarded Group and those falling into the control group. Only 158 cases in which there were complete data were included.

The first component was general, with the highest loadings on cognitive development of the child, middle loadings on family development variables and lowest on behavioural variables. The second component was bipolar and seems to contrast positive behavioural characteristics against a combination of cognitive positive social and family variables. A rotation of the axes indicates these two clusters of features more clearly. The most prominent features of the one cluster are lack of antisocial behaviour, lack of moodiness, normal activity and a tendency to regularity. The most prominent features of the second cluster are speech and language and absence of family history of developmental difficulties (see Fig. 3).

Pictorial presentation of factorial data

The clustering of features in a factor analysis can be depicted pictorially. Many clinicians find this more understandable than tables of factor loadings. In this section we provide comments on the graphs of the first and second components on the various principal components analyses described above.

Figure 1 (see first principal component analysis) The graph clearly demonstrates how features representative of specific speech delay and some non-verbal cognitive abilities cluster together, while those representative of parental and child language and social characteristics also cluster together.

Figure 2 (see second principal component analysis) The graph reveals two reasonably distinct clusters which are similar to the first.

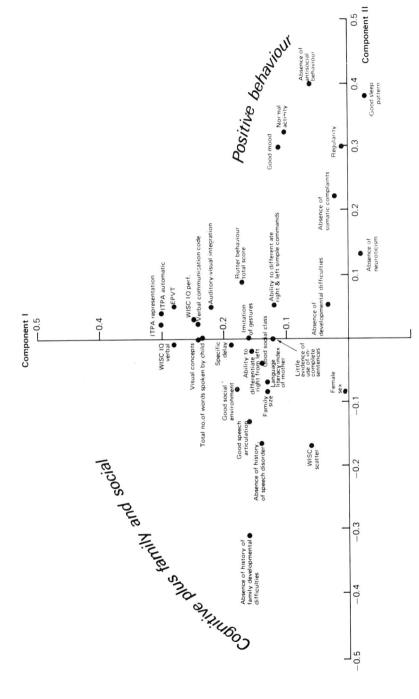

Fig. 3 Final overall principle component analysis, based on control and residual speech retarded cases

Figure 3 (see final overall principal component analysis) This graph shows how the picture becomes blurred when data from heterogeneous groups is used in a multivariate analysis. The most distinct cluster is that of behaviour. The cognitive plus social cluster is also relatively non-specific.

Discussion of findings

Those factorial findings based on the Residual Speech Retarded Group all indicate a contrast between, on the one hand, verbal ability of the child and the family and positive social influences and, on the other, uneven maturation indicated by relatively high non-verbal ability associated with specific speech delay.

Our findings provide factorial evidence of a meaningful cluster of features when analysing data from a group of children who previously had speech delay. Two of the analyses provide us with an understanding of some of the mechanisms involved in speech and language development. They lead to the suggestion that social and cultural factors are likely to be of importance in expanding verbal and communicative skills and verbal cognitive abilities, whereas satisfactory early physical development, even when accompanied by poor speech development is associated with relatively unimpaired practical abilities. Our final analysis contrasts behavioural and cognitive development.

Discriminant function analysis

Previously we have indicated that one way of classifying is to use a number of differentiating criteria in an attempt to define by dichotomization clinical subgroups within the Residual Speech Retarded Group. This is a very time-consuming and tedious exercise. Where the dependent (or predicted) variables can be sensibly or meaningfully dichotomized, so as to separate the cases into two distinct subgroups, the classical technique of discriminant function analysis has been used to ascertain which features have the greatest discriminant power. This has been used in relation to the two groups according to whether the speech delay is specific or not.

We used two sets of independent (or predictor) variables.

Set I comprised:

Behaviour—seven variables.

Cognition—WISC verbal, performance; Purdue; Frostig; EPVT; auditory visual integration; ITPA representational; ITPA Automatic; Skemp's visual concepts.

Communication—communication code; good articulation and speech of child.

Right–left differentiation difficulties—two measures.

Biological—sex.

Set II comprised:

Seven socio-familial factors and historical evidence of developmental delays in the family.

Findings (in relation to data Sets I and II above)

Specific versus general delay. The analyses indicate that the two groups can be differentiated one from the other. However, the only significant discriminant in Set I was the visual concept score (Skemp) and in Set II family history of developmental difficulties.

A note on the ability to discriminate between the right and left side of the body

It is interesting to note that the ability to discriminate between the right and left side of the body clusters with the advanced end (specific speech delay pole) of a milestone spectrum which ranges from delay of speech to delay of both speech and walking. Previously we have demonstrated that the categorization of the Residual Speech Retarded Group into specific speech delayed, intermediate delayed and general delayed groups subdivides them as well by ability on performance IQ. The question, therefore, is whether the ability to discriminate the right and left side of the body simply reflects intelligence. We explored this issue by comparing the ability (in terms of percentages) of the children in the various groups to cope first with a simple task of differentiating between the left and right side of the body (e.g. show me your right hand) and, second, a more demanding task involving crossed commands (e.g. show me your right ear with your left hand).

Our findings are of considerable interest (see Table I). In the simple task there is a steep upward gradient as one moves from the general delayed to the intermediate to the specific speech delayed group (see Table I). On simple commands the specific speech delayed group do even slightly better than the controls. These findings support the notion

Table I   *Percent of children capable of distinguishing between right and left sides of their body*

Groups of children	Simple commands	Crossed commands
	%	%
Controls	81	80
Specific speech delayed	87·5	66
Intermediate delayed	67·7	67
General delayed	45	36

that the test of right/left differences involving simple commands, in part, at least, reflects IQ. This conclusion is reminiscent of Benton's (1968) views regarding right/left discrimination and reading disability. 'When care is taken to control the variable of intelligence level, systematic study shows no important relationship between right/left discrimination and reading ability.'

However, when we come to the more demanding task of crossed commands there is a notable deterioration of performance of the specific speech delayed group. If our specific speech delayed group had previously suffered from a developmental dysphasic disorder these findings are according to expectation. It is entirely reasonable to expect some residual difficulties of comprehension which would be reflected in poorer execution of more complicated commands because the more symbolic nature of these tasks would be more difficult to comprehend. This theory would be strengthened if the pattern of deterioration held when controlling for intelligence. Without going into details we in fact controlled for performance IQ and confirmed that the deterioration is almost entirely independent of intelligence.

Conclusion

From cluster, correlational (see previous chapter), factorial and discriminant function analyses, we have evidence of the importance of language factors linking with social development, and of uneven maturation, as reflected by specific speech delay, linking with non-verbal cognitive development. Two of the major groups identified are those with general and specific speech delay. The multivariate analyses, therefore, confirm the heterogeneity even of the group of children that remains after excluding those who suffer from evident pathological disorders. Finally, our data support the notion that the group of children who previously had specific speech delay subsequently have evident language and verbal comprehension difficulties.

Part II
A Study of Hearing-impaired Children

8 The hearing-impaired child of primary school age: background factors, maternal attitudes and maternal personality

Introduction

Children with impaired hearing constitute a major group suffering from varying degrees of speech retardation. From a clinical point of view this is a clearly defined and easily identified group. It was therefore decided to broaden the research exercise by making a special study of a group of hearing-impaired children. As the prevalence of clinical deafness is under two per 1000 (Reed, 1970; Schein and Delk, 1974), it was immediately clear that Newcastle city alone was not going to provide a sample of deaf children which would be large enough to be statistically viable. In order to gather sufficient numbers we decided to accept all hearing-impaired children available, covering a slightly wider age range than we used in our parallel study of children with speech delay, and also casting the net over the whole of Tyneside rather than just the city of Newcastle upon Tyne. It must be emphasized that this group of hearing-impaired children is representative of cases known to services for deaf children in this area. As such services have been centralized we consider our group to be reasonably representative of the population of deaf children in this area, and certainly no less so than other major studies which claim to be epidemiological in nature (Freeman *et al.*, 1975).

Subjects and classification

In collaboration with a consultant paediatric otologist who provides a regional service* for deaf children on Tyneside, and also the organizers of the educational services for deaf children, a total of 59 hearing-impaired children were identified.

The hearing-impaired population consists of numerous subgroups which have to be delineated in order that interpretation of data may be valid. As with the speech retarded group, diagnostic assessments were undertaken in order to identify that group of children who could be considered as pathological deviants. These were fewer than anticipated and consisted of one severely subnormal child, three brain-damaged or spastic children and one child with a cleft palate. These five pathological subjects were not included in the statistical analyses. The mean age of the hearing-impaired sample at first assessment was eight years four months with a standard deviation of 10·9 months. We studied children with a much narrower age range, seven to ten years, than reported by Freeman et al. (1975) who included children from five to 15 years of age; our findings, therefore, are less likely to be bedevilled by variations due to age. The mean age at the second assessment was nine years four months with a standard deviation of 11·3 months. About 41% of the group were girls, 59% boys. This sex ratio is similar to that described by Freeman et al. (1975). Our cases can be included in the category of 'prelingual deafness' as the deafness almost always had an onset before the age of three years.

The 54 hearing-impaired subjects were divided into two groups:

(a) A 'profoundly deaf' group of 33 children attending the Regional School for the Deaf.
(b) A 'partially hearing' group of 21 attending various partially hearing units attached to ordinary schools in the immediate area.

The two major educational settings in which deaf children in the United Kingdom are placed are residential schools (usually on a weekly boarding basis) or day units within ordinary schools. The former have tended to cater for profoundly deaf children and the latter for partially hearing children. However, we have found that, in the north-east, the factors determining whether a child attends a unit for the partially hearing or a school for the profoundly deaf are numerous and are not based simply on extent of hearing loss. For instance, in marginal cases child behaviour, educational attainments and parental circumstances are obviously determining factors. Moreover, there is apparently no clear cut-off point of audiometric measurement which might determine the school to which a child should be admitted. It was unusual for a child to

* This is a University based unit which serves a wide catchment area.

be transferred from one school to another. A definition of deafness and audiometric data are provided in Chapter 10.

The 102 controls used in the study of speech retarded children were again used as controls for our deaf study. They were, therefore, no longer matched, paired controls but, apart from the fact that the hearing-impaired sample was significantly older, the background data suggest that they were suitable for these purposes. We were also able to compare the Residual Speech Retarded Group with the hearing-impaired group. The age difference between the hearing-impaired, the speech retarded and the controls does not affect the majority of the comparisons between them because the bulk of the tests which were administered are corrected for age and hence allow comparisons in spite of age differences.

This study is unique for two reasons. First, it is comprehensive in that it covers social, psychiatric and psychological data. Second, it has a comparison group. Several other surveys of hearing-impaired children have been undertaken by Myklebust (1964); Rodda (1970); Meadow and Schlesinger (1971) and Freeman et al (1975). Comprehensive reviews of such work have been undertaken by Myklebust (1964), Fisher (1965) and Meadow (1975). However, most of these studies have concentrated either on hearing-impaired samples of different age groups or they had inadequate control or comparison groups. The present study deals with many areas which have not previously been covered.

Aim

The aim of the present study is to obtain a clear and comprehensive picture of the total psychosocial situation, problems, resources and assets of the hearing-impaired child of primary school age in comparison to that of a child with normal hearing.

Method

As far as we can ascertain few cases escaped our net and all families proved at least partially co-operative. In all cases psychological testing of the children proved possible although only an abbreviated battery of psychological tests could be administered to some of the hearing-impaired children. For instance, only non-verbal tests could be administered to the profoundly deaf children and thus valid comparisons could be undertaken only on certain subtests.

As far as possible the same social data were collected for the hearing-impaired as for the control group. However, these data were partly retrospective in that we had to rely on case records and parental accounts. It became apparent that in some cases the earlier developmental and physical data on the deaf children were either not available or were not considered reliable. Fortunately, these cases proved to be few in number, and the amount of data available for statistical comparison was reduced by between 3–6% only, in different analyses in the case of the profoundly deaf, and by 5–10% for the partially hearing.

Results

1 Background factors and aetiology

The early development, physical and family experiences of the deaf children were investigated and compared with those of the other groups. The basic hypothesis was that the hearing-impaired children would have suffered more adverse life experiences. The results (Table I) show that this hypothesis is only partially supported. In fact, the main support for the hypothesis came from physical-organic data and associated factors like hospitalizations and the resulting separations from mother.

The following findings support the basic hypothesis:

(a) When early life developmental difficulties were summated (by giving similar weightings for each adverse experience and summing them), it was found that both study groups had a significantly higher mean developmental difficulty score than the control group. More specifically, the early sucking and swallowing of the partially hearing and profoundly deaf children proved to be significantly poorer than that of the controls, while the partially hearing had significantly more difficulty in taking solids than did the controls. The profoundly deaf group also walked significantly later than their hearing counterparts.

(b) The two study groups had many more hospitalizations and the profoundly deaf group had significantly more separation experiences from their mothers than the control group over the first three years of life.

(c) Both the study groups suffered significantly more from postnatal illnesses than their normal-hearing counterparts, and the profoundly deaf group had significantly more in the way of postnatal illness than the partially hearing group. The profoundly deaf group had a significantly higher incidence during the first five years of life of not only meningitis and measles, but also of mumps, chicken pox and whooping cough. All these illnesses, with the exception of mumps, occurred significantly more often in the first three years of life in the case of the profoundly deaf group. On the other hand, whooping

Table I Developmental, physical and associated factors—first five years of life

Feature	A = Normal hearing[b] (n = 100)	B = Partially hearing (n = 21)	C = Profoundly deaf (n = 33)	Significance A vs B	A vs C	B vs C
Difficulties with sucking and swallowing	5%	26%	23%	1%	1%	NS
Difficulty in taking solids	16%	37%	31%	NS	5%	NS
Developmental difficulties—mean score (combined category of sucking, walking, talking)	0·42	1·11	1·21	2%	1%	NS
Breast feeding: mean number of months	1·80	1·44	0·52	NS	5%	5%
Hospitalization in first 3 years	23%	47%	53%	5%	1%	NS
Major separation from mother in first 3 years	9%	11%	25%	NS	2%	NS
Measles age (years)						
0–3	32%	44%	75%	5%	1%	5%
0–5	55%	89%	94%	1%	1%	NS
Mumps 0–3	1%	5%	21%	—	—	—
0–5	17%	10%	36%	NS	2%	5%
Chicken pox 0–3	15%	33%	50%	NS	1%	NS
0–5	41%	83%	74%	1%	1%	NS
Meningitis 0–3	Nil	5%	13%	NS	1%	—
0–5	Nil	5%	13%	NS	1%	—
Whooping cough 0–3	1%	0%	14%	NS	1%	—
Mean score of postnatal infections[a]	0·77	1·56	2·5	1%	1%	2%
Convulsions	5%	14%	18%	NS	5%	NS

[a] Group mean of sum of postnatal infections.
[b] Full data only available on 100 cases.

cough was only significantly more common in the first three years of life. None of these diseases, apart from measles, occurred significantly more frequently for the partially hearing group in the first three years, but the incidence of chicken pox during the first five years was significantly greater in this group than in their hearing counterparts. However, while the profoundly deaf group had a significant excess of epileptic fits when compared to the control group, the partially hearing group did not; there were no significant differences between the two deaf groups in relation to fits.

All these significant differences emphasize the fact that the two deaf groups had encountered excesses of adverse physical-organic experiences in their early lives, and this was particularly so in the profoundly deaf. In view of the known contribution of organic factors to deafness and hearing loss, these findings are to be expected. However, they are not entirely in agreement with what is usually described in the literature, namely, that severe congenital deafness is apparently less likely than partial deafness to be associated with specific infections or diffuse brain damage. The question therefore arises in our study of whether these excesses of physical-organic illness may lead to younger children not only acquiring a severe hearing impairment but also being more seriously affected in other areas of functioning and thus being in more need of a special school for the profoundly deaf.

The profoundly deaf had also been breast fed for significantly shorter periods than the partially hearing and normal hearing subjects. This is likely to be associated with the greater frequency of physical illness in early life in the profoundly deaf group (Freeman et al., 1975).

In terms of occupational social class defined according to the Registrar General (1951), the hearing impaired had a similar distribution to the controls with only a slight excess of cases in social classes I and II. This is probably because social class I and II parents are more likely to seek treatment. Nevertheless, the lack of significant social class differences between families of hearing-impaired and control children has been reported also by Freeman et al. (1975) in his epidemiological survey. The other family and social data show a very different, more varied and complicated picture (Tables 18–20, Appendix 1). The deaf groups are by no means always worse off than the controls. There is not even a significantly greater incidence of serious deafness amongst the parents of the criterion groups (though audiometric assessments were not available and we relied exclusively on parental verbal reports). The evidence from the US National Census of the Deaf is that 'deaf' parents do not produce as a group significantly more deaf children although, of course, hereditary deafness will run in certain families (Rodda, personal communication). Only about 10% of deaf children have a deaf parent

(US Office of Demographic Studies, 1973). Our deaf groups were therefore likely to be too small for significant differences to emerge.

The following paragraphs describe areas in which either or both of the deaf groups differ significantly from the control group. As will be seen, the deaf groups have advantages over the controls in many respects.

The profoundly deaf group had significantly *less* risk in the way of adverse social and environmental experiences than either the partially hearing or normal hearing groups. There was no excess of family breakdown, family size or other family factors in the criterion groups as compared to the controls. The presence of social pathology in the families of deaf children (adverse social experiences, separation, divorce, etc.) has been extensively reported in those studies using selected samples (Farber, 1960). However, this is likely to be a referral artefact as it does not emerge when epidemiological samples are used, as in this study and that described by Freeman *et al.* (1975) in North America (see Table 18, Appendix 1).

The fathers of the profoundly deaf children are seen as significantly more satisfactory breadwinners than the fathers of the controls. A significantly higher percentage of families in the deaf groups than those in the control group regularly obtained magazines. Significantly more fathers of the partially hearing subjects belonged to a library than did the controls, but this was an isolated finding as similar percentages of mothers and children of this group and of controls belonged to a library. This contrasts with the finding that the profoundly deaf subjects were reading significantly fewer books and comics than their partially hearing and normal counterparts. Also fewer profoundly deaf subjects belong to libraries. These findings carry even more weight in view of the fact that the subjects in the deaf groups were significantly older than the controls. On the other hand, parents of both deaf groups had more reading sessions with these children than did the parents of the control group, and the differences proved statistically significant in the case of the fathers (see Table 18, Appendix 1).

A particularly interesting finding is that half of the mothers of the partially hearing were having in or out-patient treatment for 'nervousness' as against just over a third of the mothers of the controls. However, none of the mothers of the profoundly deaf reported any nervousness. The most plausible explanation for this surprising finding is that those mothers whose children attend residential schools are less subject to day-to-day stresses and strains of coping with a severely handicapped child, whereas mothers of handicapped children who attend school from home are confronted daily with the varied problems generated by such handicap.

The parents of the deaf groups appear to have on the whole more harmonious marital relationships than those of the controls: there is significantly greater agreement amongst the parents of the profoundly deaf about child-rearing practices than amongst the control parents, and the parents of both deaf groups have significantly more discussion between them on matters of health and finance (see Table 19, Appendix 1). In both deaf groups the parents have significantly more leisure outings together and the mothers of both groups also have significantly more outings on their own than do the mothers of the control group. The fathers of the profoundly deaf subjects have significantly more outings on their own than do those of the control group.

Such positive social experiences are also complemented by significantly more positive attitudes towards their deaf children in many areas. The mothers of both criterion groups made significantly more positive remarks and significantly fewer critical remarks about their children than did the mothers of the control group (see Table 19, Appendix 1).

On the other hand, the mothers of both deaf groups had significantly less in the way of regular daily verbal communication with their children than their controls, though this is to be expected (Table 20, Appendix 1). This is also true of the fathers of the profoundly deaf group. Similarly, both criterion groups of children have less interaction with their mothers than the control group. Indeed, there appears to be a gradient of communication related to the amount of hearing the child has. This tragic limitation of communication constitutes the most obvious explanation for the finding that the children of both the criterion groups confide significantly less in their parents. The contrast continues. Although the mothers of the profoundly deaf subjects have a significantly greater tendency than controls to see the importance of speech, they are significantly more inclined to use 'baby talk' than the mothers of both the hearing or partially hearing children.

The mother proved to be the one to administer discipline in 71% of the profoundly deaf subjects and in 68% of the partially hearing subjects. The corresponding figure in the control group was only 35%. This is a significant difference for both the deaf groups compared to the controls. Furthermore, management appears to be significantly more strict for the profoundly deaf with the same trend in the partially hearing, but falling just under the level of statistical significance as compared to the control group.

Additionally, parents have fewer expectations of the hearing-impaired children in spite of their being significantly older than the control group. While it is understandable that mothers of profoundly deaf children are not enthusiastic about their children going shopping (see references to Schlesinger and Meadows in the following section), there is no obvious explanation why the mothers of both hearing-impaired groups have significantly less expectation of their children tidying their own toys away than have their control counterparts. A possible explanation is that this reduced expectation simply reflects a leaning towards overprotection by these mothers.

Discussion of background factors

Considering the basic hypothesis that hearing-impaired children would have suffered more adverse experiences, it is clear from the findings that this proved to be true mainly as regards physical and organic factors.

The rest of the family and social data are more complicated. The final picture appears to be one of children whose parents are more supportive and less critical than usual, but there still appear to be a number of unexpected findings.

One might suppose that deaf children would tend to be reliant on their ability to read for acquisition of knowledge. On the contrary, we found that profoundly deaf children read fewer books and comics than their hearing counterparts and fewer profoundly deaf subjects belonged to libraries. These findings are consonant with the fact that the majority of deaf children are 'functionally illiterate' (Conrad, 1977) when they leave school. Some questions still remain. First, is it a lack of interest in reading in the home which is mainly responsible for the poor reading abilities of these children? This does not seem to be the case as more of their families received magazines and more fathers of the partially hearing subjects belonged to a library than their normal hearing counterparts. The second question is whether, despite their handicaps, the profoundly deaf are adequately encouraged to read independently by their parents. The empirical findings are that more of the parents of deaf children read to their children than parents of the normal hearing children. However, parents may not have the skills appropriate to the complex task of teaching deaf children how to read.

The third question is whether poorer intelligence and poorer hearing of our profoundly deaf children give rise to poorer motivation to achieve academically. This is likely to be a contentious issue—some authorities deny that profoundly deaf children have poorer intellectual abilities (see Chapter 10); others contend that the limited understanding of English by the majority of the deaf children is more likely to militate against the child being motivated to read independently. Some authorities have attempted to address themselves to some of these issues; for example, Lewis (1968) points out the need for recognizing the importance not only of giving deaf children 'lessons in grammar and in the regularities of the structure of English' but also of doing so 'in such a way as to maintain spontaneity of interest and some of the freshness of a living language'.

More recently, others have questioned such a view as they contend that English is by no means a living language to the deaf and that it rarely becomes so. Furthermore, Meadow (1975) asserts that there is general agreement that the young deaf child 'exposed to the difficult spoken English environment is extremely impoverished' in terms of the extent of his vocabulary and language as compared to a hearing child of equivalent age. Such proponents further argue that the deaf child's thinking, reading and writing is not in English but in patterns which are consonant with a visual mode of communication—hence English is a second language for the deaf (R. Freeman, personal communication).

Whatever the arguments, it seems that the profoundly deaf child is likely to have such great problems with understanding English that he may well not have sufficient motivation to expand his reading skills. So far the contribution of the educational system has not been discussed but, above all, educationalists must note the importance of improving the communication and language skills of the deaf. However, we believe that this is not sufficient and that improvement also has to be directed towards motivating independent reading among deaf children. Hence teachers have to seek ways of motivating the child and reinforcing academic responses. Furthermore, closer links between the school and the home could hopefully be fostered with a view to extending communicative and educational skills to the parents.

Similarly, despite the importance that they place on speech, the mothers of the profoundly deaf are more inclined to use baby talk with their children. This could be interpreted as a form of infantilization which is often an important concomitant of overprotection. Such an hypothesis is supported by the fact that the parents of the profoundly deaf have lesser degrees of expectation of their children (however, this may have multiple origins including poorer verbal communication between parents and children). The above hypothesis of overprotection is not incompatible with the findings of comparatively greater degrees of discipline imposed by the parents on their deaf children as this may simply reflect greater concern about the safety of deaf children. However, it could be argued that parents perceive their profoundly deaf children as needing to be overprotected, perhaps to an extent that could hinder their development towards self help, achievement and independence. One plausible explanation is that some of the parents of the profoundly deaf display the excess devotion, overprotection and infantilization of the syndrome described by Ounsted (1955) in relation to brain damaged children. In keeping with the theory is the evidence from Schlesinger and Meadow (1972) that parents of deaf children have a greater need to supervise their children in order to protect them. Freeman et al. (1975) also provide evidence of deaf children not being given as much independence by their parents as were their hearing controls. The fact that the fathers of deaf children take less responsibility for discipline compared to fathers of hearing counterparts, would also suggest infantilization. This finding is consonant with that of Jordan

(1962) who presents some evidence that fathers of handicapped children tend to interact less frequently with such children than do their mothers. As the subjects of the criterion groups were older than the controls it further increases the possibility of a degree of overprotection.

If this explanation is correct, then certain hearing-impaired children may be socially handicapped by their parents' attitudes. Not only may these children become retarded in their social maturity, but they also may have less meaningful communication with their parents and further be more teased and bullied. Meadow (1975) has arrived at a similar conclusion in that she suggests that parents' attitudes and child-rearing practices may contribute most to the slow development of social maturity in their deaf children.

We are not arguing that overprotection is necessarily harmful but rather that it may hamper the child's drive towards independence and social maturity. Some of our findings may be explained by an excerpt from Kallman's (1963) summary as cited by Rodda (1970):

> 'In families with both deaf and hearing children, it was reported that deaf parents tend to have more problems of control and obedience with hearing children than with deaf ones. Apparently, the deaf approach their deaf children with less uncertainty, make fewer demands of them, and have a more realistic understanding of their potentials and limitations. Towards their hearing children their attitudes are shakier.'

Perhaps hearing parents react in a similar way to their hearing-impaired and normal children.

Little in the way of comparison is possible between this and other studies on the social factors we have explored, as virtually none of the previous studies have covered the same ground. Nevertheless, it is of interest to note certain findings. For example, Myklebust (1964) found that 150 deaf children in a residential school scored approximately 15% below normal hearing children on the Vineland Social Maturity Scale. Streng and Kirk (1938) came to a similar conclusion. The implications of our findings concerning the family and social data, described above, are in agreement with the findings of Myklebust and Streng. However, as social development and language acquisition are closely interrelated (Church, 1961; Leontiev and Leontiev, 1965; Lewis, 1968) it is to be expected that children whose language development has been retarded early in life through deafness will have fewer opportunities than normal hearing children for social interaction, both within the family and outside it.

2 Maternal attitudes and personality

Apart from the measures described in section 1, the attitudes and personalities of the mothers were assessed by the Maryland Parental

Attitude Survey and the Eysenck Personality Inventory. A description of these instruments can be found elsewhere (Neligan *et al.*, 1976). As the results are essentially negative we have not provided a table.

Maryland

On none of the four scales (Disciplinarian, Indulgence, Protection and Rejection) are there any significant differences between any of the groups. At first glance this might be taken as not supporting the hypothesis advanced in the discussion of the background factors: e.g. that the hearing-impaired children are rather overprotected and infantilized. The results are, however, not necessarily contradictory. The Maryland reflects the general attitudes of mothers and tells us nothing about those attitudes which are specific to their hearing-impaired children, compared with their attitudes towards their normal hearing children. Nevertheless, it must be noted that elsewhere the Maryland differentiated between maternal attitudes of mothers of spina bifida and normal children (Van der Spuy *et al.*, personal communication). The question remains of why it discriminated in the case of spina bifida but not in the case of the hearing impaired. A precise answer is not possible, but it is feasible that, as spina bifida is a more obvious and severe debilitating and crippling condition than hearing impairment, it might have a greater effect on maternal attitudes. An alternative explanation is that the deaf children were significantly older than the controls and this might account for the lack of differences.

Eysenck Personality Inventory

On the Eysenck Personality Inventory completed by mothers we found no significant differences between the groups on the extraversion, neuroticism and lie scales.

Findings and discussion

There are few reported objective studies on the personality of parents of deaf children. This is surprising in view of the numerous studies on the psychology of the deaf child (Levine, 1956; Lewis, 1968; Rodda, 1970; Myklebust, 1964; Meadow, 1975). In a recent comprehensive study (Freeman *et al.*, 1975) 26% of the parents of deaf children were reported as having clear-cut emotional disorder but as there was no control group it is difficult to know what such a figure means. In any event, our findings tend to suggest that the personalities of mothers of deaf children are not significantly different to those of mothers of normal children.

Such lack of evidence of higher levels of neuroticism at one recent point in time does not preclude mothers from being adversely affected from time to time over the long years of having to cope with a handicapped child. Earlier in this chapter we touched on this point, where we noted that a high proportion of mothers of partially hearing children had sought psychiatric help, whereas none of the mothers of the profoundly deaf had done so. We advanced the tentative explanation for this apparently parodoxical finding that residential placement (weekly boarding) acted as a psychological buffer for the mothers against the stress of having to care for a handicapped child. Others, too, have reported that mothers of the deaf have reacted adversely to the stress of having a handicapped child, but these authors have not had the opportunity of comparing the reactions of such mothers where children have been cared for in different educational settings (Schlesinger and Meadow, 1972; Freeman *et al.*, 1975).

Much has been written about the advantages to the child of living at home while attending a special unit in an ordinary school as opposed to living as a weekly boarder in a residential school. However, little has been written about the impact on the parents of the greater or lesser sharing of the psychological burden and responsibility of caring for a deaf child. Our work suggests that the advantages to the parents of a greater sharing of responsibility with the school should not be ignored.

Conclusions

Our findings clearly demonstrate that hearing-impaired children suffered from more than the usual number of minor fevers (measles, mumps, chicken pox, whooping cough) and also major infection (meningitis/encephalitis) during the first five years of life. There was a stepwise increase in the incidence of such conditions from the normal hearing to the partially hearing to the profoundly deaf group. These illnesses usually occurred more often in the first three years of life in the case of the profoundly deaf.

No untoward degree of social and family pathology was recorded in the families of our deaf children. This is in accord with what is found in studies which generally are of an epidemiological nature, and contradicts the findings of studies using selected hospital samples.

One of the more notable findings is the lesser incidence of nervousness in the mothers of the profoundly deaf, as evidenced by the number of visits to their general practitioners, despite the greater stress of having a profoundly handicapped child than that of having a child who is partially handicapped. This is explicable in terms of the reduced exposure of such mothers to the day-to-day stresses of coping with a handicapped child, and constitutes an argument in favour of residential schooling.

The amount of communication between parents and their deaf children appears to be related to the severity of the deafness. Our data also indicate that mothers usually assume the disciplinary role, and are both more strict and supervisory and have fewer expectations of profoundly deaf children than they do of controls. This suggests an attitude of overprotection. In addition, despite the importance that they place on speech, the mothers of the profoundly deaf are more inclined to use baby talk with their children.

9 Review of the literature: intellectual and language issues

Methodological issues

It is unfortunate that the main conclusion to be drawn from a survey of the rapidly expanding literature concerning the cognitive development of deaf children is the apparent contradiction of many of the research findings; instead of the emergence of an incontrovertible body of knowledge many of the issues are still in dispute. Analysis of the methods of the studies reveals four possible reasons for these contradictory findings. First, most research has been conducted on highly selected clinical samples. Second, there has been little attempt to control for differences between hearing-impaired and control samples so that often it is not clear whether the differences found between the groups are determined by deafness or, for example, by social class differences between the groups. Third, it is essential to ensure that there are not wide differences of mean age of the groups that are being studied or of the samples of the different studies that are being reviewed. For instance, there is evidence that at younger age ranges deaf subjects may perform more poorly than their hearing counterparts on certain cognitive tests, but when the same deaf children are older one may observe a 'catching-up' phenomenon (Doehring and Rosenstein, 1960; Ross, 1966; Myklebust, 1964). Fourth, there is the task of finding or devising tests that can separately, reliably and validly tap intelligence and language. Ideally, such measures should be standardized on both the deaf and hearing subjects. In fact, the majority of tests which have been used on the hearing-impaired have been devised for the hearing, with less than a dozen tests specifically standardized on the hearing-impaired being found after an extensive search (Levine, 1971). Thus research workers wishing to study the special cognitive skills of the hearing-impaired have little alternative but to rely on measures standardized for the hearing, doing their best to select those tests considered to be least unfair to a hearing-impaired sample. Of course, such tests fall almost exclusively into the non-verbal category.

The relationship between language and intellectual processes in the deaf

The controversy: the independence or interdependence of language and thought

A major controversy among those studying deafness is whether language development is dependent on intellectual development or whether intellectual development is dependent on language. The main proponent of the view that intellectual development can proceed independently of language is Furth (1964, 1966a, 1971). The title of Furth's major work, *Thinking Without Language* (1966a), epitomizes that view. He argues that the effects of language deprivation on the deaf child's cognitive development are indirect and that adverse influences operate through impaired intellectual stimulation and motivation rather than through language deprivation. In other words, Furth models his arguments on Piaget's theory (1952, 1963, 1967) in which the acquisition of language is seen as a normal by-product of intellectual growth and as a contemporaneous form of symbolic behaviour in the child. For Furth then, language acquisition is simply a means for expressing what is arrived at independently; it is not a factor upon which thought is dependent.

In opposition to Furth there is the somewhat more popular view put forward, for example, by Lewis (1968). This is, that language and thought are complexly interrelated, and that if language development has not been allowed to take its normal course then the child's cognitive and learning development will be fundamentally affected. Such a viewpoint takes greater account of the social significance of language behaviour, which is regarded as an important source of intellectual stimulation, and of the effect it has in exercising the child's thinking processes (Luria, 1961). According to this viewpoint, the deaf child's cognitive impairment is intricately associated with the extent to which he has acquired language skills for the purpose of perceiving, understanding and describing his world.

The intellectual processes of the deaf

A variation on the theme of the controversial subject of the relationship between language and thought concerns the thinking processes of the deaf. Myklebust (1964) believes that the child who is deaf from infancy does not have the opportunity to develop fully his auditory modality and hence his perceptual processes may be established and structured differently from those of the hearing child. On the other hand, Furth (1964, 1966a, 1971) argues that the thinking processes of the deaf are similar to those of hearing subjects but that the outcome of these processes must be explained without recourse to language processes. Both of these viewpoints play down the importance of spoken aspects of language in the thinking of the deaf. Others are less convinced of the independence of intellectual processes; they emphasize the important contribution of symbolization, particularly in the sphere of language, which is considered to influence intellectual functioning (McCarthy, 1954; Whorf, 1965), even of the deaf (Lewis, 1968). Lewis (1968) points out that, while in certain circumstances deaf children may think with little or no use of language (as shown by their similar achievements to hearing children on a wide range of non-verbal cognitive tasks), in other circumstances the performance of the deaf on a range of verbal and other cognitive tasks is impaired by their inadequacy of language.

Finally, it is possible that different groups of deaf children may resort to different strategies for solving cognitive problems according to their environmental conditioning at home and at school. We can only speculate about the extent to which verbal and non-verbal symbolization contributes to the solution of any individual task. Our review of the literature leads us to conclude with other workers (Lewis, 1968; Meadow, 1975) that Furth's main hypothesis is inadequately supported not only by the work of others but also by his own data.

The importance of the environment: deaf and hearing parents

The prevalence of deaf children born to parents who are themselves deaf is usually under 10% (Rainer et al., 1969). Despite the smaller numbers in the deaf-child/deaf-parent category, comparisons of this group with the deaf-child/hearing-parent category provide an opportunity for studying the importance of the family environment.

On first principles, one could assume that deaf children of deaf parents would be at a disadvantage because of the relatively limited language resources and relative poverty of communication which might be encountered, and also because of the poorer school experiences and occupational levels achieved by deaf parents (Rainer et al., 1969). However, such theoretical assumptions are quite the opposite of what has been found in empirical research. For instance, Stuckless and Birch (1966) compared deaf pupils of deaf parents with a group of deaf pupils of hearing parents matched on age, sex, intelligence and degree of hearing impairment. The educational achievements proved superior in the case of deaf children with deaf parents. Such findings have been confirmed in other studies (Vernon and Koh, 1970, 1971; Meadow, 1968). Furthermore, they suggest that children exposed to sign language by their deaf parents very early in life, have benefited from early and systematic communication with their parents and that gains achieved through these techniques do not 'wash out' (Vernon and Koh, 1971). Apparently, these advantages occur despite the fact that deaf children of hearing parents are more likely to have exposure to pre-school nursery experiences and the opportunity for training in oral communication. The differences in educational achievement between these two groups of deaf children seem to rest on the fact that deaf parents use mainly manual communication whereas hearing parents favour oral communication.

The hypothesis put forward by some authors (Vernon and Koh, 1971) is that early manual communication is more efficient than early oral communication. This is abundantly supported by empirical research. Perhaps one of the reasons for this is that early manual communication may stimulate a form of early language development which may be more meaningful to the deaf child and appropriate to his needs, whereas in certain cases oral communication may be focusing on speech and its mechanical elements rather than on the symbolic aspects of language. More recently, Vernon (1976) has examined the controversy of oral only as compared to a combined manual and oral approach taking into account both theoretical issues and research evidence. He asserts that there are currently no advocates of the manual approach alone whereas there are still some who insist on using oral communication alone. From this review he concludes that there is strong evidence that 'total communication', consisting of combinations of oral and manual approaches and auditory amplification, that a deaf child is capable of using or profiting from, constitutes the most effective way of helping deaf children to cope with formal education, achieve satisfactory communication with their family and to adjust socially and to prepare themselves for employment. Perhaps the most telling point he makes is that it is time for the professional community to place the welfare of deaf children ahead of its personal philosophies of educational management.

Language development in deaf children

It is beyond the scope of this book to provide a comprehensive review of the complex theoretical issues concerning speech and language development in deaf children (Moores, 1972; Bellugi and Klima, 1972; Meadow, 1975; Brennan, 1976). Furthermore, as Moores (1972) has pointed out, the emergent controversies, some of which we touched on above, have often drained the energies of even the most gifted educators and researchers. In these circumstances, we decided not to be drawn into this debate and instead to confine ourselves to those basic issues immediately relevant to our research.

Moores (1972) points out that in deaf children, particularly those with profound hearing loss, the development of language is not only a different but also a more conscious and laborious procedure in which there is a heavy reliance on the visual modality. For such reasons, language acquisition of the deaf children differs qualitatively and quantitatively from the language acquisition in the hearing children. A similar view is advanced by Meadow (1975), who not only draws attention to the importance of recognizing the 'atypical' way in which deaf children acquire speech and language, but also points out that language acquisition may differ for different deaf groups according to the modes of communication used by their caretakers. She describes three main groups: (a) where (deaf) parents predominantly use sign language as a means of communicating with their deaf child; (b) where (hearing or deaf) parents simultaneously use sign and spoken English as a means of communicating with their deaf child; and (c) where (hearing) parents use spoken English as the sole means of communicating. However, even in the latter group the deaf children are subsequently likely to be exposed to peers who use sign language and so come to approximate the second group.

In the case of children with normal hearing, researchers have emphasized the importance and usefulness of internal speech in relation to the development of cognitive processes (Luria, 1961; Vygotsky, 1962; Joynt and Cambourne, 1968; Schubert, 1969). Conrad (1976) in turn poses the question of what occurs in the case of deaf children, especially those who are concurrently learning two modes of the same language, namely, speech and a sign mode? Do these children develop internal language in both modes? And if so, does the one mode help or hinder the other? Or do they develop internal language in terms of one mode only, and, if so, which one?

Meadow (1975) points out that the difficulties of language acquisition which the deaf children encounter include inner language abilities as well as the more superficial oral language skills such as speech and speech reading. Nevertheless, there is evidence that language rules are learned by deaf children in their early years and also that these rules are similar to those learned by hearing children. Furthermore, despite the method of language acquisition being different in deaf children, the vocabulary growth, grammatical complexity and syntactical structure of the language of deaf children progresses in the same way as hearing children, although such progress occurs at a slower rate in the case of the deaf (Bellugi and Klima, 1972; Meadow, 1975).

Some researchers speculate that there may be a 'sensitive period' for optimal acquisition of speech and language and that this broadly covers the first four years of life, which is when important maturational processes of a structural, biochemical and neurophysiological kind are occurring in the brain (Lenneberg, 1967; Sloan, 1967). The 'sensitive period' roughly coincides with the period of maximal rate of vocabulary growth (McCarthy, 1954) and the mastering of the fundamentals of the complex syntactical structures of language (Menyuk, 1969; Dale, 1972). Hence the concept of a 'sensitive period' implies that it is more difficult for the child to 'catch up' in those areas of language development in which he has not already achieved an appropriate degree of competence (Fry, 1966; Illingworth, 1967; Lenneberg, 1967; Meadow, 1975). For these reasons most educators attach considerable importance to general stimulation and teaching of language from the earliest years (Fry, 1966; Bellugi and Klima, 1972; Meadow, 1975; Brennan, 1976) and to the early and proper use of hearing aids (Whetnall and Fry, 1964; Fry, 1966; Reed, 1970).

Many of the above questions and arguments are academic in relation to our own research, as we had no way of reliably knowing what system of communication the deaf children were exposed to in their formative years, and, furthermore, only one of the children had deaf parents. However, our impression was that most of the children in our study did not have access to a formal sign language system in their early years of life, but that subsequently through their teachers and/or their peers such a system became a major part of their communication. As we can only speculate about the nature of the 'first language' (Meadow, 1975) of the deaf children in our study it would seem unwise to try and relate their early communication and language experiences to their later language development. All we can do is to provide a limited picture of their current language achievement.

The tests which we have used in our study on the deaf sample are standardized and the reasons for using them will be discussed below. It is necessary again to emphasize that, with one exception, the tests used did not require verbal responses for successful completion. Every effort was made to ensure that each child adequately understood the test instructions. The instructions were conveyed to the child by combinations of speech, gesture and pantomime according to the needs of the particular child.

Cognitive development

Introduction

The review of the literature that we provide below is based on research which often fails to take into account two important points. The first is that deaf children who are being tested cannot adequately use English and that the testers usually cannot adequately use sign language. The second is that tests which have been specifically standardized on hearing groups are used for comparing deaf and hearing children. The broad implication, therefore, is that cognitive studies of deaf children are open to criticisms which are similar to those about cross-cultural comparisons. In short, the criticisms concern the use of tests which may be biased in favour of one group as compared to another.

While some may argue that such tests may be unfair to the non-hearing population, the only practical way of delineating the cognitive deficits of groups of handicapped children at the time this study was undertaken was by comparing them with control groups on tests standardized for normal children. Vernon (1969) makes an important point regarding cross-cultural studies which applies equally to studies involving comparisons between hearing and deaf groups. He says 'the main problem in testing groups with diverse backgrounds is, not to find a culturally unbiased test, which is impossible, but to find tests from which safer inferences can be drawn.' We have attempted to take this message into account both in reviewing the research literature and in the tests used in our own study. We have as far as possible confined ourselves to a range of tests which are not dependent on the modality in which the children are handicapped and which allow for their successful completion.

Verbal and non-verbal abilities

The most consistent finding in research on the deaf is that their mean verbal IQ is usually significantly below that of their hearing counterparts. However, in terms of non-verbal IQ, the mean scores of groups of deaf children lie within the normal range but tend to be slightly below average (Murphy, 1957; Vernon, 1968; Wiley, 1971; Myklebust, 1964). A characteristic picture has emerged in different studies of differences between verbal and performance scale IQs of hearing-impaired children, with better results on the performance scale—such as that of Hine (1970) who examined a representative sample comprising 100 partially deaf children, aged 8–16 years, on the WISC. The mean verbal IQ proved to be 82 and the mean performance IQ 98.

There is also evidence that the intelligence of deaf children is not static and their IQ tends to become normal with age. From an analysis of the test results of the Wechsler Bellevue Scale, Myklebust (1964) reports that, from the ages 14–20, both the verbal and the performance IQs of deaf children have improved. Furthermore, by the age of 20 the children's better scores on the performance scale had compensated for the poorer scores on the verbal scale sufficiently to raise their global score to near normal. Lewis (1968) infers from this that the intelligence of the deaf tends to be retarded in its development rather than permanently impaired.

Although it is likely that the more adversely affected the child's hearing, the greater will be his disability in dealing with verbal tests, this does not necessarily mean that there is a simple linear relationship between audiometrically measured hearing loss and verbal IQ (Lewis, 1968). Indeed, verbal achievement is influenced by other factors, such as educational influences in the home and school, in addition to auditory impairment and, as Meadow (1975) has argued, the fundamental handicap of the deaf is not of hearing but rather of language. Nevertheless, in general it is evident that hearing loss impedes the child from scoring as high on verbal as on non-verbal tests.

Specific disabilities

In this section we turn our attention to various specific types of cognitive functioning in which deaf children are alleged to show impairment. This is a complex area where precise definitions and sharp psychometric tools are not readily available. The situation is complicated by the fact that we are dealing with maturing processes and their organization, and these are continuously being influenced and modified by experience. In an attempt to bring some order into this rather untidy area some researchers have elected to use models of intelligence to explain the wealth of findings of cognitive impairment of the deaf. The best known of these is Myklebust (1964) who attempts, by a *tour de force*, to explain his findings as well as those of others in terms of Guilford's (1959) theoretical model of intelligence, by focusing on Guilford's five types of mental operations, namely, cognition, memory, convergent and divergent thinking and evaluation.

Although Myklebust's approach is interesting it has some serious theoretical limitations which are beyond the scope of this chapter. We have therefore preferred to consider a number of more conventional concepts in relation to the cognitive abilities of the deaf and without being tied to any theoretical model. We will concentrate, therefore, on the specific abilities of memory, perception and conceptual thinking.

Memory

There is some evidence (Levine, 1963; Lewis, 1968; Furth, 1971) that even where deaf and hearing children have been matched on factors such as age, non-verbal IQ and social class, the deaf tend to perform worse on certain tests. For example, it has been found that the deaf are less successful than their hearing counterparts with certain types of memory span. Withrow (1968) reports poorer visual memory for successively presented sequences of stimulus material though not for simultaneously presented sequences. Similarly, Goetzinger and Huber (1964) found that deaf children had poorer delayed recall but similar immediate recall when compared with hearing children. In a study by McCarthy and Marshall (1969), in which a deaf and a hearing group were compared with regard to visual recall of objects placed to the right and left according to a particular order, the deaf children did significantly worse. On the other hand, Blair (1947) found that on the Knox Cube Test for visual memory span the deaf performed significantly better than their hearing peers. In a cross-sectional study by Furth (1961), the visual memory of deaf and hearing subjects in two ranges, 7–10 years and 11–12 years, was tested. There were no significant differences between the deaf and hearing in the 7–10 year age range, but in the 11–12 year range the hearing children were markedly better. Furth suggests that the inferiority of the older deaf children might be attributed to a deficiency in training and experience. Conrad (1973) raises the possibility of other even more complex determinants which involve the question of different coding strategies. He found that in a group of deaf subjects who were all prelingually deaf some scored better than a hearing group on a test of short-term memory. The evidence showed that this subgroup of deaf subjects used a speech coding strategy in contrast to the visual coding strategy which is predominantly used by most deaf subjects.

Clearly, some of the findings on memory are contradictory. Whether factors such as experience and training, or perhaps age or a particular type of coding strategy constitute the important determining influence on the findings is difficult to say. A longitudinal, as opposed to a cross-sectional approach to the study of memory impairment of the deaf might possibly provide a clearer picture.

Perception

In other studies in which tests of visual perception have been used it has again been found that the deaf do worse than their hearing peers on some tests but not on others. For instance, Myklebust and Brutten (1953) compared a deaf and a hearing group on tests of pattern discrimination and pattern recognition and found that the performance of the deaf was significantly poorer than that of the hearing children. Carrier (1961), on the other hand, observed no significant difference between a deaf and a hearing group on a test where they had to associate colours with weights. Such studies are relevant to a debate of whether deaf children compensate for their impaired auditory sense modality by utilizing other sensory modalities. Investigations of the ability of deaf and hearing children to use tactile cues have often proved contradictory. In a study by Schiff and Dytell (1971) it was found that deaf and hearing children did not significantly differ in their ability to identify letters by touch. Blank and Bridger (1966) also found no significant differences between a deaf and a hearing group on a cross-modal task. However, Larr (1956) compared deaf and hearing subjects on the Marble Board Test, a picture test and a tactile motor test and found that the deaf were better than or equal to their hearing peers.

Conceptual thinking

Studies of the conceptual thinking of the deaf have been more challenging, mainly because of the difficulty of finding or devising tests which are appropriate and valid. Nevertheless, there are studies which have highlighted some important relevant factors.

First, it should be emphasized that while perceptual and conceptual abilities inevitably overlap, it is nevertheless important for practical purposes to attempt to distinguish between them. One important difference is the degree to which abstract symbolic thinking is necessary to cope with the test; tests of conceptual ability tend to be typified by the greater degree of abstract/symbolic thinking (Rosenstein, 1961; Pettifor, 1968).

Pettifor (1968) compared the conceptual ability of 59 'hard-of-hearing' and 59 normal hearing children (matched for sex and age and with similar mean IQs) by a sorting test which required cards to be grouped according to certain similarities or differences. The performance of the 'hard-of-hearing' group proved significantly poorer and resembled that of younger normal children. A number of investigations have been carried out by Furth and his colleagues in which Piaget-type tests have been used to study the conceptual ability of the deaf (Furth and Youniss, 1965; Youniss and Furth, 1969). In one of these studies (Furth and Youniss, 1969) a group of deaf adolescent boys of above-average IQ (Wechsler performance IQ range 111–125; age range 13–19 years) were each tested on six individual non-verbal Piaget-type tasks which involved the principles of 'formal operations' (for example, judgement of displaced volume; probability, judgement of three-dimensional space, etc.). Furth and Youniss found that none of the deaf subjects succeeded consistently on all tasks and also that the concept of conservation of volume and of probability proved particularly difficult for the deaf to master. Although no comparison group of hearing subjects was used, it is important to note that Furth's group of subjects was generally older than the age at which hearing children would normally have acquired the concept of formal operation (Flavell, 1963; Bruner, 1964). Our interpretation of these findings is that the stage at which certain conceptual skills are evident is later in deaf than in normal hearing children. Furthermore, there is evidence that deafness does not equally affect all abstract reasoning processes. For instance, as Meadow (1975) has pointed out in her summary of some of Furth's earlier studies, deaf children show relatively little retardation in concepts of sameness and symmetry but have obvious difficulty in grasping the concept of opposition.

Interim discussion

In view of the various factors such as the problems of sample selectivity, age and the 'catching-up' phenomenon and test validity, caution must prevail when generalizing about the specific cognitive disabilities of the deaf and when attempting to explain and interpret them. Nevertheless, the weight of evidence supports the view that the deprivation of sound and its concomitant effect on language and other experiences tends to impose certain constraints on the deaf child's flexibility of thinking. The effect is that of comparative disability or impairment in certain areas of cognitive functioning, and in particular in those areas in which there is a greater demand for abstract thought.

This is not to say that the deaf are incapable of abstract thought, or alternatively that their thinking is of a 'concrete' nature. On the contrary, there is evidence that there is as reasonable potential for abstract thought among the deaf as there is among the hearing (Furth, 1966a; Lenneberg, 1967; Vernon and Miller, 1973). On the other hand, the evidence also suggests that higher levels of conceptualization, although not totally dependent on verbal functioning, appear to be facilitated by such functioning (Lewis, 1968; Chovan, 1972; Conrad, 1973; Meadow, 1975). In summary, while there is agreement that the deaf are capable of abstract thought and that they have relatively normal non-verbal intelligence there is disagreement as to how well the deaf cope in relation to certain abstract/symbolic tasks as compared with their hearing peers.

Educational attainment

Deaf children have also proved to be educationally retarded both in respect of reading ability, and in terms of progress with age, in reading

(Wrightstone *et al.*, 1962). The annual reading gain per year in terms of reading age is less than 12 months and therefore the absolute amount of educational retardation increases with age (Meyerson, 1963). Findings from the 1971 large-scale testing of academic achievement of the deaf under the auspices of the US Office of Demographic Studies (1973) have shown that deaf children show better achievement in reading in their first three years of schooling than in their later schooling, but after the early years tend to do better in spelling and in arithmetic than in reading. Nevertheless, it is evident that the academic achievements of these children are poorer than those of hearing children, and, furthermore, that the rate of improvement after the age of 12 years is particularly slow. There is the view, however, that these cognitive and educational handicaps are more often an indictment of the educational system than an inevitable consequence of deafness (Vernon, 1969, 1976). This suggests that greater effort is needed on the part of teachers of the deaf, and that more research into teaching techniques is necessary in order to find better ways of helping the deaf to realize their full academic potential at an earlier age than is apparently possible at present.

While in England concern has been expressed about the ability to teach deaf children to read (Watson, 1967), there has been little in the way of empirical studies of the relationship between extent of hearing loss and reading attainment. More recently Conrad (1977) has presented his findings on a study of the reading ability of deaf school leavers aged 15–16½ years. He reports that reading is significantly affected by degree of deafness and by level of non-verbal intelligence. He points out that if adequate reading is represented by a reading age of nine years only half of his deaf sample, regardless of their extent of their hearing loss, fall above this cut-off. Furth (1966b) adopts a more stringent criterion of a functionally useful ability to read which is achieved at about 11 years of age. Conrad points out that if this criterion is used then 75% of his sample would be considered as lacking adequate reading skills. He concludes that the reading performance in England and Wales is very similar to that of American children with both deaf populations reading very poorly.

Factor analysis

Factor analysis can be undertaken on full (verbal and non-verbal) cognitive data of a partially deaf population but not on that of a profoundly deaf population because valid assessment of verbal abilities of the profoundly deaf is not possible. One of the few reported studies of factor analysis of a partially deaf population is that of Hine (1970). He administered a battery of tests, which included the WISC to a partially deaf sample of 100 children age 8–16 years, and carried out a factor analyses on 24 variables. He found three important factors which he described as verbal ability, numerical ability and performance ability. A separate analysis on the WISC subtest data revealed the same three factors. This finding, as Hine claims, is in contrast to factor analysis of the WISC on normal populations in which only two main factors—verbal ability and performance ability—were found (Maxwell, 1959; Silverstein, 1969). Hine suggests, on the basis of his findings, that verbal, numerical and performance abilities tend to develop relatively more independently in partially deaf than in hearing children.

Summary

This briefly summarized review suggests that childhood deafness will constrain and hamper both language and cognitive development. In fact, there is ample evidence that the cognitive impairment is selectively concentrated on verbal abilities, as the deaf child population has much the same distribution of non-verbal intelligence as the general population (Murphy, 1957; Ives, 1967; Vernon, 1968; Myklebust, 1964; Wiley, 1971). Such selectivity is highlighted by the finding that deaf children's verbal IQs are affected more than their performance IQs with a mean discrepancy of 30 points in some studies (Lewis, 1968). However, even on certain non-verbal tasks, particularly those that require abstract skills, deaf children perform significantly less well than hearing children. It seems that the greater the level of abstraction needed for the task, the more likely it is that the deaf child will fare worse than the hearing child (Pettifor, 1968; McCarthy and Marshall, 1969), but this comparatively poorer performance on such tasks lessens with age.

Of crucial importance is the relationship between intelligence and language. Furth (1964, 1971) is of the view that thinking and cognitive processes can develop without the benefit of verbal language. However, the most common view is that if verbal language is impaired, cognitive development and learning will also be impaired (Oleron, 1953; Blank, 1965; Lewis, 1968; Myklebust, 1964). The situation is made even more complex by the fact that the deaf are not a homogeneous group. Not only are there different types and also different degrees of severity of deafness, but also differences in the age of onset. In most studies only a few of such factors have been considered. Without a detailed description of the sample it is difficult, therefore, to know how to interpret and assess findings.

Finally, it is necessary to comment on some of the other factors which are particularly likely to affect the cognitive functioning of the deaf. For instance, in certain cases the same brain pathology that caused the deafness could also have caused the cognitive impairment. Other factors which have to be taken into account include the type and severity of deafness, the different modes of communication and language acquisition to which the deaf children have been exposed in their early years, hereditary factors and general quality of family life and social environment.

Implications for our research

With the above review in mind, the four main factors which could distort the picture obtained during our research are as follows:

(a) *Representativeness of the sample* As already stated, we believe our sample is as representative and typical of a total population of deaf children in a community as those used in any of the other major epidemiological studies.

(b) *Controlling for differences* between the groups of hearing-impaired and control children. Research workers have considered two main differences:

(i) *Social class factors.* In a previous chapter we point out that there is no significant excess of social and family pathology in our hearing-impaired sample as compared to the controls. Hence, any differences that emerge are unlikely to be determined by such factors.

(ii) *Intervening experiences.* The main intervening factors are whether the deaf child has a deaf parent and the type of communication used at home and at school. It is usually found that less than 10% of deaf children have deaf parents. This proved to be the case in our study where only one child (approximately 2%) had parents with a severe degree of deafness. As our sample tended to be small and as we wanted it to be representative, we did not exclude even that single case described above.

(c) *Measures used* While we agree that none of the measures used have been designed specifically to tap abilities of hearing and deaf children without being reliant on the hearing modality, we have confined our attention to those tests or subsections of the tests which we consider to be more appropriate for comparing deaf and hearing children. The problem with tests specifically designed for deaf children is that, with a few major exceptions (e.g. Drever and Collins), they are insufficiently standardized for age and/or have not been satisfactorily revised. In addition, insufficient experimental work has been carried out on these tests in relation to other types of handicap, and also with normal hearing children of different ages. In these circumstances we decided to use well recognized standardized tests which have been widely used on deaf populations and, furthermore, to use only those subtests which we felt would be relevant for the deaf.

10 The hearing-impaired child: intellectual and educational development

Introduction and aim

The aim of this part of the research was to study the intellectual, language and educational development of those hearing-impaired children who were not suffering from severe multiple handicaps. Of the 59 subjects who were identified as hearing-impaired, five had severe multiple handicaps and were accordingly excluded from psychological assessment. The mean age of the hearing-impaired group was eight years four months at first assessment and nine years four months at the second assessment. We compared this group with a normal control group of 101 children, whose salient characteristics have already been described. In addition, in certain analyses we have included a comparison group of 84 speech retarded children who had had no serious organic problems or intellectual handicap and who were of the same age as the control group. As the psychological literature is so central to an understanding of our findings we have reviewed it more comprehensively than is usual in the previous chapter.

Method

Selection of cases

Our initial intention was to match the hearing-impaired with the speech retarded and the normal controls with regard to the variables of sex, age and, broadly, social class. This proved to be impossible as the prevalence of clinical deafness is under two per 1000 (Reed, 1970). We therefore sought a statistically viable sample by accepting for inclusion all available known hearing-impaired children from a slightly wider age range and from a wider area than the immediate Newcastle city boundaries. In fact, we sought out children living in the geographical area of Tyneside. The mean age at first assessment was seven years five months for the controls, seven years six months for the speech retarded and, as already stated, eight years four months for the hearing-impaired. The age differences do not affect the comparisons as only age-corrected tests were used. The sex ratios of the groups were, however, similar. Furthermore, there were no significant occupational social class differences between the control and hearing-impaired groups.

Tests used

As Reed (1970) points out verbal tests of intelligence are not valid with deaf children. We therefore confined ourselves *mainly* to the use of those tests which were non-verbal:

(i) *Conceptual maturity* The test used was the Goodenough-Harris Draw-a-Man Test (1963).

(ii) *Psycholinguistic performance* The tests used were the non-verbal items of the Illinois Test of Psycholinguistic Abilities (1968).

(iii) *Visuomotor perception* The test used was the Frostig (1966).

(iv) *Non-verbal intelligence* The performance items of the Wechsler Intelligence Scale for Children (1949) were used.

(v) *Reading* The Schonell Graded Word Reading Test (1960) was used.

Definition of deafness

In a physiological sense deafness implies a significantly reduced sensitivity to sound; psychologically it refers to an inability to adequately hear and perceive speech and other meaningful sounds (Watson, 1967; Schein, 1968). There are, of course, varying degrees of deafness. Children with such hearing impairment are usually classified as profoundly deaf or partially hearing in terms of a number of important criteria in addition to the most obviously important, namely, response to audiometric measurement.

Audiometric assessment of our hearing impaired group

It is important to distinguish between those children who are profoundly deaf and those who are partially hearing. We were able to subdivide our hearing impaired sample according to whether the children were attending schools for the profoundly deaf or units for the partially hearing. The factors determining attendance at one or other type of school were not simply those of severity of hearing loss (see Chapter 1), though degree of hearing was an important consideration. In marginal cases, child behaviour and parental circumstances were often the deciding factors and therefore there was a certain degree of overlap. Using these crude criteria 33 of the 54 children were classified as profoundly deaf and the other 21 as partially hearing. From Fig. 1 it will be seen that the average hearing loss for our profoundly deaf group is just beyond 80 decibels and that our partially hearing group is about 68 decibels. Hearing loss of around 80 decibels or more is considered by many (Reed, 1970; Moores, 1972; Vernon, 1976; Conrad, 1977) to distinguish those with profound deafness from those with less severe degrees of deafness. Hence we believe that the criteria we have used for defining profound deafness are satisfactory. However, this may not be so in the case of our partially hearing group. An examination of our audiometric profile reveals that the greater proportion of our partially hearing group falls towards the more severe end of the hearing loss continuum. It is therefore possible that some of those whom we have included in the partially hearing group might be considered as seriously deaf by other research workers. Furthermore, it needs to be noted that we have used the terms profound deafness and partially hearing as if there was a clear-cut distinction between them whereas it is evident that hearing loss lies along a continuum. We appreciate that the dichotomy we have used is a relatively simple one, but its purpose was to allow a study of the effects of different degrees of deafness.

Findings

Differences between the means of the groups on cognitive tests

From Table I it will be seen that on all measures used the performance of the total hearing-impaired group is significantly inferior to that of the control group. The least differences occurred on the WISC performance scale and the widest differences on the Draw-a-Man, Frostig visuo-perceptual, and on the non-verbal ITPA tests. Furthermore, though the differences between the WISC performance quotients of the deaf and controls was only 4 points, the difference between these two groups on the Schonell is 14 points. It is therefore evident that the hearing impaired are seriously retarded in reading.

Of considerable theoretical importance is the fact that the mean scores of the total deaf group are closer to those of the Residual Speech

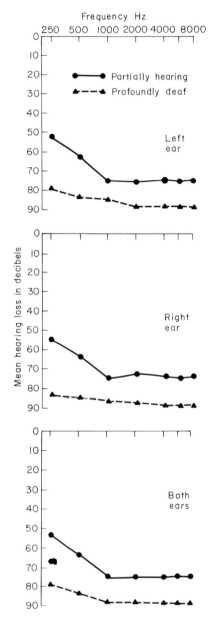

Fig. 1   Mean hearing loss in decibels at each frequency for partially hearing and profoundly deaf groups

Table I *Comparisons of total hearing-impaired and control groups on cognitive and educational data*

		Groups			Significance	
Tests		A = Controls	B = Residual speech retarded	C = Total hearing impaired	A *vs* C	B *vs* C
Draw-a-Man	m	96·4	92·4	89·3	1%	5%
	s.d.	9·9	9·1	8·9		
ITPA (visuomotor tests)	m	31·4	28·7	28·4	1%	NS
	s.d.	3·4	4·0	3·2		
Frostig	m	95·9	86·8	82·5	1%	5%
	s.d.	11·9	14·1	9·6		
WISC performance	m	101·2	94·9	96·8	5%	NS
	s.d.	11·0	13·3	13·1		
Schonell	m	93·9	80·4	79·5	1%	NS
	s.d.	19·2	15·7	12·4		

Draw-a-Man: Conceptual maturity standard score; ITPA: Mean scaled score for five non-verbal tests; Frostig: Visuo-perceptual Quotient; WISC: Non-verbal Intelligence Quotient; Schonell: Graded Word Reading Quotient.

Table II *Degrees of deafness and intellectual and educational development*

Test		A = Controls (n = 101)	B = Residual speech retarded (n = 84)	C = Partially hearing (n = 21)	D = Profoundly deaf (n = 33)	A vs C	A vs D	C vs D	B vs C	B vs D
Draw-a-Man	m	96·4	92·4	91·4	88·0	1%	1%	NS	NS	1%
	s.d.	9·9	9·1	10·1	7·9					
ITPA (visuomotor tests)	m	31·4	28·7	29·8	27·4	NS	1%	1%	NS	NS
	s.d.	3·4	4·0	2·9	3·1					
Frostig	m	95·9	86·8	83·4	81·9	1%	1%	NS	NS	NS
	s.d.	11·9	14·1	8·9	10·0					
WISC performance	m	101·2	94·9	101·9	93·6	NS	1%	5%	5%	NS
	s.d.	11·0	13·3	11·8	13·0					
Schonell Graded Word Reading	m	93·9	80·4	87·6	74·4	NS	1%	1%	NS	1%
	s.d.	19·2	15·7	13·7	8·3					

Significance

NS = not significant

Retarded than to those of the controls. Furthermore, in two instances, namely, the Draw-a-Man and Frostig visuo-perceptual tests, the mean scores of the total hearing-impaired group are significantly lower than those obtained by the Residual Speech Retarded Group.

When data is re-analysed according to the degree of deafness (Table II) the partially hearing group prove to be superior to the profoundly deaf group on all the tests and significantly so on three of the tests. The profoundly deaf group are significantly inferior to the controls on all the tests used but the partially hearing are significantly inferior to the controls on only two of the five tests (i.e. in terms of conceptual maturity and visual perception). Furthermore, the partially hearing group are significantly superior to the Residual Speech Retarded Group on the performance IQ.

Subtest profiles

So far the hearing-impaired group as a whole has proved inferior to the control group on the WISC performance scale and the summated scaled score of the five ITPA non-verbal subtests. The next question is whether such inferior performance is general or whether it is specific to certain subtests (and conversely whether the deaf perform better on any of the subtests). The data is more simply presented in profiles.

On the ITPA Profile (Fig. 2) it is evident that the scores of the hearing-impaired are significantly depressed on four of the subtests compared to the controls, but on manual expression they score significantly better than the Residual Speech Retarded Group. This subtest was devised to measure the ability of the child to express ideas by means of manual gesture and pantomime. Therefore the circumscribed better ability on the test is likely to represent greater exposure, experience and training in the use of a manual form of communication. Another interpretation of these findings is that this better ability of the hearing-impaired represents a better inner language potential than is revealed by the other subtests. It is therefore evident that, with one exception, the abilities of the hearing-impaired as a whole group as found on the ITPA are poorer than those of the controls, even in those tests which are considered non-verbal.

The ITPA Profile in Fig. 3 includes separate profiles for the partially hearing and profoundly deaf groups. It clearly shows that the profoundly deaf have the superior score on manual expression but their other ITPA abilities are below those even of the Residual Speech Retarded Group and significantly so in the case of visual reception and visual closure. The shape of the profile of the partially hearing group is similar to that of the controls but is slightly depressed. This suggests

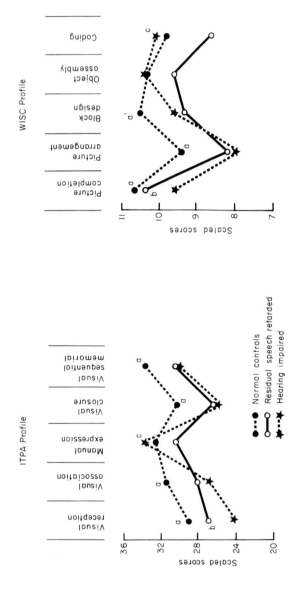

Fig. 2 (left) ITPA non-verbal mean scaled scores of hearing impaired, residual speech retarded and control groups. a = controls significantly better than hearing impaired at 0·001 level; b = residual speech retarded significantly better than hearing impaired at 0·01 level; c = hearing impaired significantly better than residual speech retarded at 0·001 level.

Fig. 4 (right) WISC non-verbal mean scaled scores of hearing impaired, residual speech retarded and control groups. a = controls significantly better than hearing impaired at 0·01 level; a¹ = controls significantly better than hearing impaired at 0·05 level; b = residual speech retarded significantly better than hearing impaired at 0·05 level; c = hearing impaired significantly better than residual speech retarded at 0·001 level.

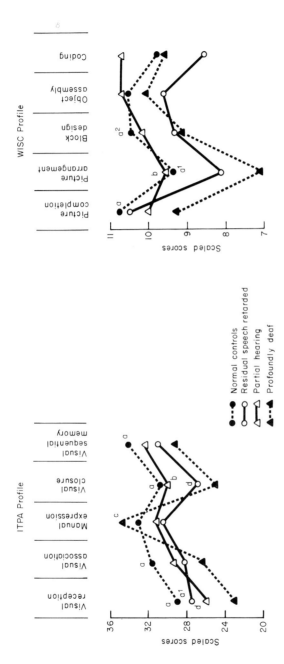

Fig. 3 (left) ITPA non-verbal mean scaled scores of partially hearing, profoundly deaf, residual speech retarded and control groups. a = controls significantly better than profoundly deaf at 0·01 level. a¹ = controls significantly better than partially hearing at 0·05 level; b = partially hearing significantly better than profoundly deaf significantly better than partially hearing than controls at 0·05 level, profoundly deaf significantly better than residual speech retarded at 0·01 level, profoundly deaf significantly better than partially hearing at 0·01 level; d = residual speech retarded significantly better than profoundly deaf.

Fig. 5 (right) WISC non-verbal mean scaled scores of partially hearing, profoundly deaf, residual speech retarded and control groups. a = controls significantly better than profoundly deaf at 0·01 level a¹ = controls significantly better than profoundly deaf at 0·001 level; a² = controls significantly better than profoundly deaf at 0·05 level; b = partially hearing significantly better than profoundly deaf at 0·01 level, partially hearing significantly better than residual speech retarded at 0·05 level.

that the non-verbal skills of the partially hearing are generally similar to those of hearing children. Of equal importance is the similarity of their profile to the Residual Speech Retarded Group. This is not surprising as varying degrees of language impairment are common to both of these groups. In the case of the Residual Speech Retarded Group, evidence suggestive of language delay is provided in an earlier part of this book, and in the case of the deaf the evidence derives from the literature.

The findings on the manual expression task of the ITPA are important. The task consists not only of manual gesture but also how to manipulate specified objects (Paraskevopoulos and Kirk, 1969). It therefore tends to tap more concrete aspects of expressive communication. The better ability of the deaf on manual expression is to be expected in view of the greater experience in this form of communication. Such experience is less likely to be obtained with less severe degrees of hearing loss where verbal communication is more likely to predominate.

On the WISC performance subtests the profile of the hearing-impaired group (Fig. 4) is significantly depressed on picture completion, picture arrangement and block design, compared to the controls. This is not the case for object assembly and coding. Reed (1970) considers that the subtests of picture arrangement and picture completion are more verbally loaded and thus the inferior scores of the hearing-impaired group on these two tests is according to expectation. Similar explanations cannot be offered for block design.

When the hearing-impaired group is divided into the profoundly deaf and partially hearing it is immediately evident that the WISC performance subtest (Fig. 5) profiles of the partially hearing and the controls are broadly similar. The profile of the Residual Speech Retarded Group is similar but depressed in comparison to the controls. The profoundly deaf are particularly poor in relation to the controls on the two subtests which are thought to be verbally loaded (picture completion and picture arrangement) and only on coding does their mean score approach that of the controls.

Subtest scatter

The standard deviation of the subtests of the WISC and the ITPA were used to derive measures of scatter. The means and standard deviation of the subtest scores of each child were calculated and the standard deviations thus obtained were used as a measure of scatter. These standard deviations were themselves summed, group by group, and the mean standard deviation scores for each group were then compared.

Subtest scatter was not calculated for the profoundly deaf group as they were not given all the tests. The partially hearing group obtained a significantly greater (p <0·001) subtest scatter than did the controls for both the WISC and ITPA.

Deafness and specific intellectual functions

To what extent subtests of tests such as the WISC and ITPA reliably measure specific cognitive functions is debatable, as each subtest usually requires more than one intellectual function for it to be completed successfully (Cohen, 1959; Rappaport *et al.*, 1968; Hine, 1971; Hare *et al.*, 1973). Nevertheless, it is customary to attempt to identify the main cognitive function measured by that subtest. Such definition allows a cautious interpretation of deficits or strengths displayed by groups of children with a particular disorder. While Cohen (1959) generally advises against interpretation of individual subtest scores, Sattler (1974) is of the view that cautiously made interpretations may prove to be useful. This is a view which appears to be shared by Kirk and Kirk (1971) in relation to the ITPA and by Glasser and Zimmerman (1967) in relation to the WISC.

In the light of the above the following attempt at interpreting individual subtest scores must be seen both as tentative and speculative, but nevertheless aimed at generating hypotheses which might be tested in other research.

Visual perception

On tasks where visual perception plays an important part, e.g. on the ITPA subtests of visual reception and visual closure, the profoundly deaf group had significantly poorer results than their hearing counterparts. Similarly, on the WISC subtests of picture completion and block design, the profoundly deaf group again proved to be significantly inferior to the hearing group. In contrast, the partially hearing group fared significantly worse than their hearing counterparts on only one of the above subtests, namely, visual reception of the ITPA; on the other hand, the partially hearing were superior to their profoundly deaf counterparts on visual association.

The studies already quoted in the review section of the previous chapter provide contradictory evidence on the subject of the visual perceptual ability of the deaf. In our study the profoundly deaf group show wide impairment in visual perceptual ability compared with the controls both in terms of global and subtest scores. In the case of the partially hearing group, it is less widespread, being evident only on the visual reception subtest of the ITPA and on the global score on the Frostig Test of Visual Perception. The differences in visual perceptual ability between the profoundly deaf and partially hearing groups in comparison with their normal hearing counterparts leads us to the view that it is determined by the degree of deafness of the different subgroups. It has been claimed that different sensory modalities can take over in the face of a serious impairment in one of the other modalities. However, our findings do not provide evidence in support of the view that there is widespread compensation in visual perceptual ability of deaf children.

Conceptual thinking

We have already noted that the evidence in the literature tends to support the view that the cognitive abilities of the deaf are more likely to be adversely affected on tasks dependent on abstract and symbolic thinking. We have examined the subtests, and two of them in particular appear to require greater degrees of non-verbal reasoning ability of an abstract nature. On the WISC the non-verbal subtest which has been found in research to relate significantly to an analytic conceptual ability is picture arrangement (Kagan *et al.*, 1964; Sattler, 1974). On the ITPA by definition the visual association subtest demands an ability to comprehend the relationship between visually presented symbols and hence emphasizes the child's ability to cope with analogies (Paraskevopoulos and Kirk, 1969). It is evident that both these tests have additional perceptual components but this is the kind of overlap to which we have already referred. It is to be noted that on both of these subtests the profoundly deaf group have significantly poorer results. These findings are consistent with evidence in the literature as reported above. On the other hand, the partially hearing did not significantly differ from the controls on these two subtests. We therefore conclude that degree of hearing loss is related to extent of deficit on abstract and symbolic abilities.

A third non-verbal test which, in our view, falls into the conceptual thinking category is the manual expression subtest of the ITPA. Not only does it measure the child's ability to express ideas by means of manual gesture and pantomime, but it also demands a degree of symbolic thinking for its execution. On this test the profoundly deaf group scored significantly better than the control, Residual Speech Retarded and partially hearing groups.

Memory

Only one task was administered to our hearing-impaired subjects in which memory could be said to be the predominating function. That was the visual sequential memory subtest of the ITPA.

On this subtest the profoundly deaf group proved to be significantly poorer than the controls, whereas the partially hearing group did not significantly differ from the controls. It would be unwise to advance a general conclusion about the deaf child's memory function on the basis of this subtest alone. On the other hand, our findings of the poorer performance on visual sequential memory is consistent with Withrow's (1968) findings. He found that his deaf group did worse on tests of visual memory for successively presented stimulus material and where non-meaningful visual forms, which are also characteristic of the ITPA visual sequential memory subtest, featured. It may well be, as we have already argued, that degree of hearing loss is an important factor which contributes to the cognitive differences we have found between the partially hearing and profoundly deaf, compared to the normal controls.

Discussion

There is general agreement that hearing loss and its associated effect on language tend to limit the hearing-impaired child's modes of thought (Lewis, 1968; Rodda, 1970; Myklebust, 1964; Meadow, 1975). Our findings provide evidence in support of this view, and also give rise to a number of other conclusions which are of considerable importance. Perhaps the most notable of these is that cognitive impairment appears to be related to the severity of hearing loss. Second, the partially hearing group showed minimal cognitive impairment on non-verbal tests and indeed on only one of these was there a significant difference from the controls. This may well be a chance finding as most of the other major studies do not report any such impairment. Third, a widespread pattern of cognitive impairment was found in the case of the profoundly deaf; however, this group of children did particularly well on the manual expression subtest of the ITPA, which is a measure of gestural language. This better performance may merely reflect a greater degree of experience in gestural language which is a commonly used form of communication among the deaf (Levine, 1960).

Correlation of handicaps and achievements

One simple way of re-analysing our data is to develop an index of handicap in four main areas in relation to all the groups which we have so far studied in this research. For the purposes of this analysis we have included the two subgroups of speech retarded children defined and

Table III　*Evidence of handicap*

Handicap	Control group	Specific speech delay group	General delay group	Partially hearing group	Profoundly deaf group
Hearing[a]	1	1	1	3	4
Language[b]	1[d]	2[d]	2[d]	3[d]	4[d]
Speech dealy[c]	1	3	3	3	4
Motor delay[c]	1	1	3	1	2
Total handicap score	4	7	9	10	14
Rank of groups	1	2	3	4	5

[a] Based on global audiometric assessment
[b] Based on clinical assessment by speech therapist
[c] Based on early history
[d] Weighting system: clear evidence = 4; moderate evidence = 3; minimal evidence = 2; no evidence = 1.

described in an earlier section of this monograph. The two groups are the specific speech delayed group (i.e. those with speech delay but whose walking milestones were achieved early) and the general delayed group (i.e. those whose speech and walking milestones were both delayed). We have arbitrarily given weightings of 1 to 4 to each of the groups on the basis of historical or clinical evidence (see Table III). The handicaps which we have identified as important are hearing as assessed audiometrically, language as assessed by the speech therapist, and speech and motor delays as based on historical evidence. In Table III we have arranged the groups so that they range from that with the lowest total handicaps score, which is the normal control group, to that with greatest handicaps score, which is the group of profoundly deaf children.

We then advance the hypothesis that the group with highest loadings of handicaps will have the lowest cognitive achievements and vice versa. We can now test this hypothesis by comparing handicapped scores with cognitive achievements. In Table 21, Appendix 1, we provide the mean scores of the ITPA subtests for the five groups which we have studied. We also provide rankings of the scores of these subtests, which immediately allows us to compare these rankings with the sum of ranks on the index of handicap. When we compare the bottom two rows of this table it is evident that our hypothesis is only broadly substantiated, with the partially hearing group doing far better and the general delayed group doing much worse than would have been forecast by our hypothesis. This unexpectedly good performance from the partially hearing may be a reflection of the handicaps incorporated into the weighting system (three hearing and speech and only one motor).

With regard to the subtests, the pattern described above is usually repeated. The only variations of note are that the control group is worse on manual expression and visual closure than predicted by our hypothesis; and the profoundly deaf are far better at manual expression than expected.

When this analysis is repeated using subtests of the WISC (Table 22, Appendix 1) we perceive the same pattern—the general delayed group doing far worse and the partially hearing far better than we would have expected. Indeed, on this occasion the partially hearing (in terms of their sum of ranks) do even better than the controls. Returning to the subtests, the specific speech delayed group do better than expected on only one subtest and worse than expected on all the others. The profoundly deaf do better than expected on object assembly and coding. These general patterns and trends are repeated on the other tests used, namely the Frostig Test of Visual Perception, Draw-a-Man Test of Conceptual Maturity, WISC performance IQ and the Schonell Graded Word Reading Quotient (Table 22, Appendix 1).

Such analysis can only indicate trends as it relies on rankings and not statistically significant differences. Nevertheless such trends become important if they persistently emerge on a variety of cognitive tests. Our findings lead us to conclude that children with milder degrees of deafness compensate for their handicaps on non-verbal tests by doing as well as the specific speech delayed group on the non-verbal tests of the ITPA and as well as the controls on the performance subtests of the WISC.

The next most obvious pattern is the poor performance of the general delayed group, as on no subtest do they perform better than expected. We again conclude that the poor performance of this group is determined by general intellectual backwardness. The profoundly deaf do badly on most subtests, but despite their heavy weighting of handicap they perform especially well on manual expression of the ITPA. It is worthwhile noting that the profoundly deaf also do better than expected on object assembly and coding, while the specific speech delayed group do worse than expected on these two tests (in terms of rank order). This demonstrates that in certain areas the profoundly deaf, either through compensatory adjustment to their hearing loss or through experience and training in related skills, are able to function almost as well as their hearing counterparts.

Finally, it is interesting to note that a far better prediction of outcome on the basis of handicap could have been obtained by using a smaller selection of indices of handicap. For instance, the use of speech and motor milestones alone would have predicted performance on cognitive tests better than the index which we have actually used (see Table III).

Rank order and gaps between non-verbal subtests (WISC and ITPA)

WISC

In a previous chapter we described an alternative way of studying the data by comparing the rankings of the mean scores on the subtests of the groups studied. The rankings are shown in Table IV. It will be seen that on the non-verbal scale of the WISC the rankings of the partially hearing and profoundly deaf groups are similar to each other but appear very different from those of the controls. After ranking the mean subtest scores and using the Newman-Keuls Test for correlated data and testing for a significant gap we found that there were no significant gaps between any of the subtests in the case of the partially hearing group; on the other hand, in the case of the profoundly deaf there was a significant gap between object assembly on the one hand and picture arrangement on the other (p <0·01). This is repeated in relation to coding, picture completion and block design and on all occasions this consisted of a significant gap with picture arrangement (p <0·01).

In summary, in terms of rankings of the non-verbal subtests the partially hearing and profoundly deaf have similar patterns, but only the profoundly deaf have a number of significant gaps on the WISC.

ITPA

The exercise described above was repeated for the ITPA subtests. The differences in patterns of rankings are not as evident as in the WISC. It will be seen that, with some minor variations, the patterns of rankings of both the partially hearing and the profoundly deaf are similar to each other and indeed also similar to those of the controls (see Table IV).

When comparing subtest scores with each other within groups it will be seen that, in the case of the partially hearing group, the only significant gap was between visual reception and visual sequential memory (p <0·05). However, in the profoundly deaf group the gaps between manual expression and the remaining subtests are all significant (p <0·01). In addition, there are significant gaps between visual sequential memory and visual reception (p <0·01), visual closure (p <0·01) and visual association (p <0·05).

In summary, in the ITPA tests the pattern of rankings of the non-verbal subtests for the three groups are broadly similar. However, when testing for a significant gap using the Newman–Keuls Test a wide scatter is found in the results of the profoundly deaf group. This is almost entirely determined by the better performance on the manual expression subtest, compared with the other subtests. However, the

Table IV   *Rank order of mean scores on non-verbal subtests of ITPA and WISC*

	Controls	Partially hearing	Profoundly deaf
WISC			
Picture completion	1	4	3
Block design	2	3	4
Object assembly	3	1·5	1
Coding	4	1·5	2
Picture arrangement	5	5	5
ITPA			
Visual sequential memory	1	1	2
Manual expression	2	2	1
Visual association	3	4	3
Visual closure	4	3	4
Visual reception	5	5	5

High rankings e.g. 1, 2 = high achievements
Low rankings e.g. 4, 5 = low achievements

profoundly deaf also do well on the visual sequential memory test compared with the results on the remaining subtests. We discuss elsewhere the patchy performance of the partially hearing group as measured by scatter. As scatter was determined by verbal as well as non-verbal tests we were unable to apply this technique to the profoundly deaf group. However, the present test for significant gaps between subtests in a sense also reflects scatter, and it is evident that this is greatest in the profoundly deaf (as measured by non-verbal subtests). This patchy performance of the profoundly deaf is unlikely to be determined only by deafness or its causes. It is more likely to be affected by an interaction of aetiological factors, severity of deafness and environmental influence. This appears to be less true of the partially hearing who, in many ways, function more like the control group than like a deaf group.

Verbal abilities of partially hearing children

Introduction, aim and method

In the previous section we gave an account of the intellectual and educational progress of partially hearing and profoundly deaf children. There we confined our analyses to those tests which were non-verbal (with the exception of the reading test) as it is usually not possible to obtain valid results on verbal tests with a significant percentage of deaf children.

Nevertheless, a subgroup of the deaf sample, consisting of 17 of the 21 partially hearing children, were able to complete all the verbal tests. The findings on these tests enable us to study the verbal abilities and handicaps of this highly selective group of hearing-impaired children. In this section we therefore address ourselves to an analysis of the verbal items of the verbal scale of the Wechsler Intelligence Scale for Children (WISC) and the five main verbal subtests of the Illinois Test of Psycholinguistic Abilities (ITPA). In addition we compared the partially hearing group both with the controls and with the group of children who were previously speech retarded and described as the Residual Speech Retarded Group (see earlier chapters).

Findings

Our findings are simple. They consist of the demonstration of a gradient on all subtests from controls to speech retarded to partially hearing. While the children in the partially hearing group show a significantly poorer performance than the controls on every subtest, the difference from the Residual Speech Retarded Group is significant on only six of the ten subtests studied (see Tables 23 and 24, Appendix 1) and on four of these the differences are on language subtests.

Discussion

The interpretations are again simple—the majority of partially hearing children have a manifest potential for developing certain verbal abilities while the profoundly deaf do not. Nevertheless such achievements of the partially hearing are more limited than those of a group of children with handicaps of speech but virtually none of hearing. These findings are consistent with the hypotheses advanced in the previous section, namely, that the greater the evidence of handicap in the areas of hearing and speech, the poorer the language and cognitive achievements of the child (see Table III).

It is notable that the highest mean score on the WISC verbal subtest is on arithmetic, which resembles the findings by Hine (1970) with his partially hearing sample. He claims that this improved performance is a reflection of the fact that some non-verbal skills are involved in the solution of the items in this subtest. These findings suggest that the more one can enhance the child's hearing through artificial aids the greater the likelihood of increasing the child's intelligence and attainments. Perhaps the most important conclusion from this analysis is that the greatest handicap of deaf children, even when the deafness is not profound, is the area of language (Meadow, 1975).

Principal component analysis

A principal component analysis was undertaken on cognitive data from the total hearing-impaired, Residual Speech Retarded and control group subjects (Fig. 6). The variables included were of the non-verbal type listed in the methods section, the exception being the Schonell Graded Word Reading Test. Only the first two components were considered meaningful:

    (i) Component I accounts for 36% of the variance. A study of the loadings on this first component reveals that it has reasonably

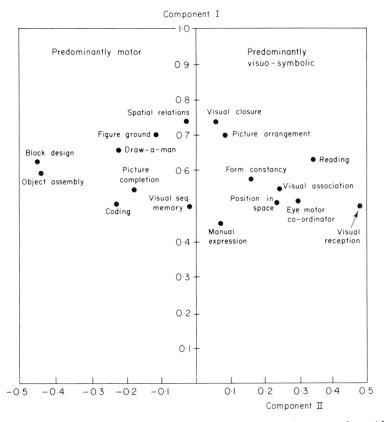

Fig. 6 Principal component analysis of cognitive data for control, residual speech retarded and deaf groups

high positive loadings on all variables included in the analysis. We therefore view it as a general component of intelligence. This is to be expected as this is precisely the type of data which was included in the component analysis.

(ii) The second component is bipolar and accounts for 6·8% of the variance. At the one pole are variables predominantly representative of motor tasks and the pole has been labelled thus. At the other pole are tasks which are predominantly visuo-symbolic in nature and the pole has been labelled visuo-symbolic representation (see Fig. 6 and Table 25, Appendix 1).

From Table 25, Appendix 1, it will be seen that on components I and II the deaf group have a significantly lower score than the controls. On component II the score of the deaf is significantly inferior to that of the Residual Speech Retarded Group. The inferiority of the deaf on what we have described as a non-verbal general component merits explanation. It is possibly because even so-called conventional non-verbal tests may contain verbal elements. This is consistent with Myklebust's (1964) view of non-verbal tests—he argues that it is wrong to regard all non-verbal tests as equally non-verbal because it is likely that some of these tests involve considerable ability of the type commonly referred to as verbal. Reed (1970) also supports this view.

If the mean component scores provided in Table 25, Appendix 1, are located on the map of Fig. 6 then the deaf group would fall into the lower left quadrant of the component map (i.e. negative scores on both the first and second components) and thus lean towards the motor pole. The control group would fall into the opposite positive quadrant and lean towards the visuo-symbolic representation pole. The Residual Speech Retarded Group would fall into the lower right quadrant, i.e. a slight leaning towards visuo-symbolic representation.

This technique of combining cases from three different groups for the sake of component analysis may be open to the criticism that multivariate techniques can be applied only to data from the same population: however, this view is not unanimous (Cattell, 1965).

Interim discussion

It is clearly evident from our results that the overall performance of our hearing-impaired children falls below that of the normal hearing control children on all the cognitive tests administered. The exceptions to this general trend will be discussed later. The finding that the total hearing-impaired group's performance on a non-verbal IQ test falls significantly below that of the control group is only broadly consistent with most of the earlier findings on the deaf. In our view the differences between the findings are likely to be determined by the selectivity of the sample studied. If we had taken only a profoundly deaf sample we would have ended with a jaundiced view of the cognitive ability of deaf children. Indeed, our finding underlines the importance of studying as representative a sample of the hearing-impaired population as possible. This leads to the following conclusion.

Our own results certainly do not support the conclusion that the hearing-impaired obtain scores comparable to the normal hearing population, despite the use of non-verbal performance tests. Possible explanations are as follows:

1 The deaf constitute a heterogeneous group of disorders and the findings of different studies will, in part, reflect this heterogeneity. Different findings may therefore reflect differences in the groups under scrutiny. For instance, there is evidence that the cognitive abilities of deaf children of deaf parents are likely to be less impaired than deaf children with hearing parents (Meadow, 1968). We were not confronted with this complication as only one of our deaf children had deaf parents.

2 Our subjects were younger than those of most of the reported studies. The evidence suggests that the achievement by the deaf on intelligence tests is age-related, that inferiority compared to normal hearing individuals will tend to disappear by the age of 20 and that at the age of 20 the deaf actually score above average on performance items like picture completion, object assembly, block design and digit symbol (Myklebust, 1964). As our subjects are younger than those involved in previous similar studies, the effects of their hearing impairment on their intellectual functioning could well be more marked than is seen in studies using older subjects. We can therefore argue that the deficit on the WISC performance tests shown by our sample could well disappear with age. This younger group should provide us, however, with more information about the earlier effects of hearing impairment on intellectual development.

Educational attainment

The low score of the profoundly deaf group in comparison with the control, Residual Speech Retarded and partially hearing groups (Table II) is consistent with the findings of other research workers (Wrightstone *et al.*, 1962; Meyerson, 1963; US National Demographic Study, 1973; Conrad, 1977). It is of interest to note the gradient which consists of the control group having a mean reading quotient in the 90s, the Residual Speech Retarded and the partially hearing groups mean reading quotients in the 80s and the profoundly deaf group a mean reading quotient in the 70s. Furthermore, a glance at Table 22, Appendix 1, shows that the general delayed group has a mean reading quotient which is similar to that of the profoundly deaf group. Our conclusion must, therefore, be that the partially hearing group is only slightly impaired on educational attainment in terms of reading quotient, as compared to the controls, but that the profoundly deaf group is seriously retarded.

It has often been assumed that the poorer academic functioning of deaf children in residential schools for the deaf, as compared with deaf children in special classes in ordinary schools or in integrated classes in ordinary schools, is determined by three main sets of factors: first, living in a special environment away from normal home conditions; second, isolation from the verbal and social stimulation which is usually available in ordinary school from one's normal peer group; third, the selection of the deaf children for residential education on the basis of multiple handicaps. While it is tempting to suggest that the poorer educational attainment of our profoundly deaf group has been determined by their residential educational environment it should be remembered that their poor attainment is consistent with the pattern of findings on other cognitive tests, and also that the educational attainment of our deaf group has been based on a reading test which is essentially a verbal test. Hence, a more likely explanation for the poor attainment of the profoundly deaf group is that it is mainly a function both of the severity of deafness and of the multiplicity of handicaps which are commonly found in deaf children in residential settings.

Finally, as recently pointed out by Meadow (1975), the relationships between eduational functioning, school environment and family variables are complex and, indeed, there may be important interaction effects between such variables. For instance, she has demonstrated that residential schooling appears to be associated with more favourable functioning on certain tasks in the case of deaf children of deaf parents as compared with deaf children of hearing parents.

Some final comments

Explanation of handicaps in terms of models of intelligence

After a penetrating analysis of the structure of the main models of intelligence, Hearnshaw (1975) concludes,

'The pioneers in the scientific study of intelligence, Spearman, Burt and others, endeavoured to replace faculties by statistically established factors, and this endeavour has persisted to the present day, and to the elaborate factorial structure proposed by Guilford (1967). These endeavours, though an advance on faculty psychology, have not, however, been wholly convincing.

There is an element of arbitrariness in factorial solutions, and it would seem that unless the questions are posed, and the measure selected, on the basis of much more penetrating theory about the nature of intelligence, factorial analysis cannot provide convincing answers.'

Our own results suggest that the use of any one model of intelligence is too narrow for a meaningful interpretation and understanding of the complexities of cognitive functioning of deaf children. The factorial structural model has been useful for the interpretation of certain patterns but for others a teleological type of explanation of an appropriate adjustment to a 'silent' world is more meaningful. A similar approach can be advanced in relation to an understanding of cross-cultural differences in intellectual performance (Vernon, 1969). The implication of this is that man will use his intelligence to adapt to any personal limitations and environmental constraints as exemplified by the high ability on manual expression of the profoundly deaf.

The study of the intellectual performance of the deaf has had a long history, while the study of the intellectual performance of the culturally deprived and minority groups is of comparatively recent origin. The deaf child and culturally deprived child in fact have much in common, because the deaf child is basically deprived. He is deprived of language and the normal exposure to sound and speech and the wealth of information which the normal child usually obtains through his auditory modalities. In addition, he is subject to the negative attitudes confronting any minority group in our culture, and further, his intellectual and educational performance is consistent with that of children of minority groups (see Jensen, 1969; Jencks, 1972). Our background data suggest that he might be deprived of all the more adventurous explorations indulged in by hearing children. We would like to suggest that the poorer performance of a child from a different culture or deprived environment can be seen in the same light as the poorer performance of the deaf child. On the one hand, his poorer performance may be due to non-exposure or limited exposure to certain life experiences, intellectual games and language to which the average child in our culture is subject, and, on the other hand, he may perform worse on some tasks because they do not tap abilities which are meaningful to his particular existence.

Husen (1975) claims, 'different socio-cultural settings vary in the demands they make on intelligence. They not only require different amounts but chiefly different kinds of intelligence. Consequently, each social context demands and trains just the variety of intelligence that is needed for that particular setting.' This view sheds some light on our own findings. Our profoundly deaf children are superior in manual expression because their social context demands and trains that variety of their intellectual ability which is needed for their particular setting. However, as they grow up and become more integrated in the main stream of our culture, it becomes increasingly necessary for them to improve their ability to cope with and manipulate abstract symbols. This is a complex subject which goes beyond the brief of this book.

Considering that we are in most cases dealing with very early deprivation in the deaf, it certainly supports the arguments by investigators such as Clarke (1968) and Kagan and Klein (1973) that the effects of even severe early deprivation may not be reversed without concentrated effort. Society provides intensive help in the form of special schools, specialized teachers and small classes, available from an early age to school leaving age in an attempt to overcome the effects of that deprivation. The earlier impressions of favourable outcome associated with pre-school compensatory programmes have now been put into a less optimistic but more balanced perspective by empirical research. Hence while one would support such a lobby to promote pre-school programmes for deaf children, the authoritative conclusions (Bronfenbrenner, 1976) regarding the effectiveness of such programmes in the case of underprivileged children have important implications in the case of hearing-impaired children.

Cerebral dysfunction

On the basis of our biographical and psychological assessment a case could be made for the existence of an important degree of cerebral dysfunction in our hearing-impaired sample, particularly in the profoundly deaf group. In a previous chapter we described excesses of major postnatal illnesses in the profoundly deaf group compared with the controls. The same was true for epileptic fits. While the partially hearing had some excess in comparison to the controls these were usually not significant. The other evidence in support of a cerebral dysfunction hypothesis derives from psychological testing. At its best this is usually 'soft' and indirect evidence (Birch, 1964). In our study the psychological evidence available is mainly from the use of the Frostig Developmental Test of Visual Perception on which children with varying degrees of brain damage have been found to show a marked paucity of performance (Maslow et al., 1964, p. 497).

Both our hearing-impaired groups scored significantly worse than their normal counterparts on the Frostig Test, and the partially hearing group had a significantly higher scatter than the controls on the subtests of both the WISC and the ITPA. The subtest for the profoundly deaf group on the WISC and ITPA has not been calculated because only the non-verbal subtests could be administered to this group. Superficially, our findings might be considered as supportive evidence of cerebral dysfunction in our hearing-impaired groups. However, such evidence is weakened by doubts about the validity of the Frostig Developmental Test of Visual Perception as a psychological indicator of cerebral dysfunction. Corah and Powell (1963) factor-analysed the Frostig and found it to tap little more than general intelligence and chronological age. Their findings appear to refute the claim that five separate perceptual factors are measured by the Frostig. It is for this reason that we have concentrated only on the overall Frostig score in this project: while some clinicians might interpret the lower scores on the Frostig as evidence in support of significant cerebral dysfunction amongst our hearing-impaired subjects, we would not give very much weight to this evidence. Furthermore, though the high subtest scatter might be suggestive of cerebral dysfunction, it might also merely indicate that the hearing loss has affected their performance on certain subtests to a greater extent than on other subtests. While the same arguments in favour of an organic hypothesis apply to the interpretation of some of the subtest scores on the WISC performance scale, it must be emphasized that even here (see Table 22, Appendix 1) the general pattern of subtest scores bears little resemblance to patterns which are clinically considered to be characteristic of cerebral dysfunction.

Nevertheless, we cannot ignore the fact that organic factors are often important causes of deafness. Nor can we ignore the possibility that cerebral dysfunction may have contributed to the poorer performance of our hearing impaired group, particularly the profoundly deaf, but we have no way of estimating the extent of this contribution.

Conclusion

As a group, the hearing-impaired children performed significantly worse than their normal counterparts on the vast majority of the non-verbal cognitive tests. But it would be an oversimplification, if not erroneous, to conclude that hearing-impaired children of junior school age are 'less intelligent' than normal hearing children. It is more helpful to consider the hearing-impaired in terms of their cognitive strengths and weaknesses. A more meaningful overall summary is provided by a study of the principal component analysis where a pattern emerges which is consistent for each component. The first component measures general intelligence and on this the controls do best, the Residual Speech Retarded Group obtain an intermediate score and the deaf do worst. On the second component, which is a bipolar dimension of 'visual symbolic ability versus motor ability' the mean score of the hearing-impaired group falls at the motor pole, that of the controls at the visual symbolic pole and the Residual Speech Retarded Group in between. Such findings suggest differences in cognitive style between the groups of children. We believe that these findings reflect a difference of learning strategies between deaf and hearing children, with the former responding to readily observable, manipulable and meaningful stimuli and the latter coping more comfortably and spontaneously with the more abstract type of tasks. It is not the first time that researchers have concluded that the deaf learn more through doing and seeing than through speaking and hearing. However, we do not see this as absolute as we do not deny the value of helping the hearing-impaired to make maximum use of residual hearing and/or oral communication, however elementary.

Such comments ignore the fact that the deaf are not a homogeneous group. We have used one simple classification, namely, the division of the hearing-impaired into profoundly deaf and partially hearing subgroups. Indeed, the patterns elaborated above are much more typical of the profoundly deaf than of the partially hearing. In many ways, the partially hearing resemble the normal control group while the profoundly deaf almost always have a significantly depressed cognitive profile compared to that of the controls. However, the other major characteristic of the profoundly deaf group is the patchiness of the pattern of their subtest scores. This is most clearly highlighted on the ITPA where the profoundly deaf have a subtest score higher than all the other groups studied. Thus while profound deafness adversely affects most cognitive functions, it would seem that certain functions may actually be enhanced on the one language ability where hearing loss is no impediment because the mode of communication used can be considered to be a variant of sign language and is therefore more meaningful to the deaf child. Nevertheless, our findings suggest that hearing loss makes an important contribution to the poorer intellectual functioning of hearing-impaired children.

This appears to contrast with the findings of Conrad (1977) who found 'no significant effect of hearing loss on non-verbal intelligence'. We have examined his data and it is clear that there is an overall trend in the same direction as we have found in relation to extreme degrees of hearing loss. Even so, account needs to be taken of certain important differences between the two studies. The deaf sample in Conrad's study were school leavers aged 15–16½ years and so were much older than our sample. We have already acknowledged (p. 167) the possibility that the significant effect of hearing loss on the intellectual functioning of our deaf groups could well be more marked than is the case in studies using older subjects. Furthermore, Conrad has only used the Raven's Progressive Matrices Test (1960) whereas we used a wider range of non-verbal tests which included the WISC performance scale. In our study the pattern of cognitive impairments is consistent across the tests we used and this leads us to consider that our findings are valid for this younger age range.

We were also able to study the functioning of the partially hearing group on verbal subtests of the WISC and the ITPA (in contrast to the profoundly deaf group who could not validly complete such tests). On the subtests the partially-hearing invariably fared significantly worse than the controls but this pattern was not as consistent in relation to the Residual Speech Retarded Group. The one surprising finding is that the partially hearing group, despite usually doing worse than the specific speech delayed group on verbal subtests, are better at reading.

In this chapter we also provided evidence that the functioning of handicapped children is related to the number and severity of their handicaps. The most obvious impediment of hearing-impaired children is deafness but such children are also likely to suffer from degrees of brain damage and intellectual impairment. These handicaps are inter-related and it is no easy task to tease out the importance of the direct and interactive effects of each of these in relation to later performance. Our findings lead us to take the stance advanced by Lewis (1968) that language and thinking are complexly interrelated in contrast to the view of Furth (1966a, 1971) who sees language and thought as largely independent.

In conclusion, the finding that the cognitive test scores of our deaf sample are depressed, might lead to the erroneous conclusion that deaf children of primary school age are simply 'less intelligent'. Such a conclusion would be an oversimplification and is belied by the fact that our results indicate that, while profound deafness widely affects most cognitive functions, certain intellectual abilities may in fact be enhanced, with the profoundly deaf scoring better than their hearing counterparts. For instance, the profoundly deaf performed significantly better than their normal hearing counterparts on the one language ability test where hearing loss is no impediment, namely, the 'manual expression' subtest of the ITPA. In contrast, those with some hearing, i.e. the partially hearing subjects, in general obtained a pattern of scores which is similar to that of the normal hearing sample.

11 The hearing-impaired child: behaviour and personality

Introduction and review of previous literature

There are few systematic studies of psychiatric disorder, behaviour or temperament of deaf children. Most of those undertaken are marked by inadequacy of the research design or lack of appropriate instruments or both and therefore it is not surprising that the findings are often ambiguous, inconclusive or contradictory and certainly not comparable.

Further, the validity of the earlier research into maladjustment of deaf children was seriously diminished by the fact that these were mainly paper and pencil tests which took little account of the children's poorer educational achievements and poor language developments (Reivich and Rothrock, 1972). The findings of such research were, in brief, that hearing children proved more well adjusted than deaf children and that deaf children raised in families where other members were deaf proved better adjusted than those raised in families where the other members were not deaf (Myklebust, 1964).

Two other features which merit comment are those listed by Vernon (1961) in his account of brain-injured deaf children; these are psychological immaturity and denial which children used as characteristic defence mechanisms. Treacy (1955) also concludes from his research that deaf children are less socially mature than hearing children. Furthermore, there is some evidence that, during adolescence, the social maturity of seriously deaf children tends to decrease while that of partially hearing children tends to show an improvement (Treacy, 1955). Myklebust (1964), from studies using the MMPI and his recent review, concludes that the level of social maturity of deaf children is some 10% poorer than that of hearing children and that this, rather than maladjustment, is their major psychological handicap. Levine and Wagner (1974) report on their use of a projective technique called the 'Hand Test'. From their work they attribute the problems of deaf individuals to frustration in the face of their speech and language difficulties.

More recently, test instruments which are completed by teachers or parents have found favour. Their strength is that they are dependent on objective observations and not on the self-reporting of the deaf. While their validity for the deaf has not as yet been adequately established they provide a useful means of comparing the reported behaviour of deaf and non-deaf children.

One instrument which has been used quite extensively is the Bristol Social Adjustment Guide (Stott, 1963). Fisher (1965) compared 83 hearing-impaired children aged five to 16 with a control group and found that the hearing-impaired were significantly more withdrawn than the controls. On the other hand, Rodda (1970), using the same instrument, reported a percentage of deaf adolescents who were disturbed which was only slightly greater than that of controls. Unfortunately, the size of his control group was too small to inspire confidence.

There is also the question of whether factorial analysis will reveal distinctive behavioural patterns in terms of the structure of the factors that are found with deaf children as compared to normal children. Reivich and Rothrock (1972) undertook factorial analysis of the behaviour of 327 deaf students aged six to 20 using the Behaviour Problem Check List (Quay and Peterson, 1967) which is completed by teachers. Their first two factors were structurally similar to those which have been described in all factorial studies and have been labelled conduct and personality or neurotic factors (Kolvin et al., 1975). Their third factor, which they describe as 'immaturity inadequacy', has been described in only a few studies such as that of Quay and Peterson (1967) and is likely to be an artefact of the wide age range of children studied or of the features included in the factor analysis. None of these factors are therefore specific for the deaf. Their fourth and fifth factors account for so little of the variance that it seems reasonable to ignore them. This decision is supported by the large number of variables (55) included in the analysis. Of greater importance is the fact that the means for the above three factor scores prove to be very similar to those of normal elementary school children but very significantly lower than those found with institutionalized delinquents. The only interpretation that is therefore possible on this factorial analysis is that the behaviour of deaf students is little different from that of their hearing counterparts. However, such findings must be viewed with caution as the mean age of the deaf is very much higher than that of the normal children with whom they are being compared and as far as can be ascertained no allowance has been made for age.

Another question is whether greater degrees of deafness are associated with higher rates of maladjustment. Bowyer et al. (1963) found little difference between the severely deaf and partially hearing using the Bristol Guides. Rodda (1970) also reports that the degree of hearing loss does not appear to be correlated with the extent of maladjustment.

The prevalence of psychiatric disturbance among deaf children has been variously estimated from less than that found in the general population to significantly higher. Simpson (1964) reports an 11·7% rate of maladjustment among 359 deaf school children aged 15 to 16. No figures are provided for controls so it is difficult to know what these figures represent. Williams (1970) cites an estimate, by the National College of Teachers of the Deaf, of 6% at the age of 12 years but again this was an uncontrolled study. In addition, he has undertaken an analysis of the types of psychiatric disorder in deaf maladjusted children and concludes that these are similar to those found in normal children and in children handicapped in other ways. He found that approximately 44% had antisocial disorders, but only 8% had neurotic and 10% mixed disorders. Other disorders which were diagnosed with reasonable regularity were psychosis in 20% and hyperkinetic disorders in 10%. As with children without hearing impairment, the main association is with disturbed home backgrounds.

Aim

The aim of this chapter is to survey two groups of hearing-impaired children, namely, partially hearing and profoundly deaf, in relation to their behaviour and temperament as described by parents and by their teachers.

Method

The assessment instruments used were the Temperament Scale (Garside *et al.*, 1975) and the Behaviour Scale (Kolvin *et al.*, 1975). These instruments and their various dimensions have been described in previous chapters. The Teacher-Child Scale B (Rutter, 1967) was also completed for each child.

Findings

Rutter Teacher Scale (see Tables I and II)

When the deaf group is divided into profoundly deaf and partially hearing groups (Table I) the high rate of behavioural disturbance of the

Table I Classroom behaviour and severity of deafness—mean scores—teacher's questionnaire (Rutter Scale 'B')

Feature	A = Control	B = Residual speech retarded	C = Partially hearing	D = Profoundly deaf	A vs C	A vs D	B vs C	B vs D	C vs D
Rutter total	5·8	8·3	7·3	12·0	NS	1%	NS	5%	5%
Antisocial subscale	1·1	1·7	1·6	3·4	NS	1%	NS	1%	5%
Neurotic subscale	1·4	1·6	1·1	1·8	NS	NS	NS	NS	NS

Table II Classroom behaviour—psychiatric abnormality: Rutter questionnaire in percentages

	A = Controls	B = Residual speech retarded	C = Partially hearing	D = Profoundly deaf	chi-squared		
					B vs D	C vs D	A vs D
Score 9+	18	36	28	54	5%	1%	1%

profoundly deaf is revealed. In the Isle of Wight Study it was found that, of the children finally diagnosed as showing psychiatric disorder, 53% scored above the cut-off point of 9, compared to 7·1% of the general population (Graham and Rutter, 1970, p. 158). In a subsequent study Rutter and colleagues (1975) report a slightly higher percentage (10·6%) of the population on the Isle of Wight Study falling above the designated cut-off while the percentage (19·1%) in an Inner London borough was almost double that of the Isle of Wight Study. In our study many more of our controls scored above the cut-off of 9 as compared to the Isle of Wight child population figures and, indeed, our figures are more similar to those reported in the Inner London borough. It is of interest to note that the percentage of our controls who scored above the cut-off is double that of the Isle of Wight Study, the percentage of our partially hearing group is three times higher, while that of the profoundly deaf is about six times higher (see Table II). Our results show that neither the controls nor the Residual Speech Retarded Group differ from the partially hearing. On the other hand, the profoundly deaf group differ significantly from the controls and the Residual Speech Retarded Group on both the mean total score and mean antisocial subscores of the Rutter Scale. From Table I it will be seen that there are no significant differences between the groups on the neurotic subscore of the Rutter teacher questionnaire. Furthermore, it is evident that the most seriously disturbed group is the profoundly deaf and this disturbance is mainly of an antisocial variety.

Behaviour Scale—Based on an interview with mother (see Tables III and IV)

Both hearing-impaired groups showed less behaviour deviance on overall assessment, but this was statistically significant in the case of the profoundly deaf only (see Table III). Of the nine dimensions studied (neurotic, antisocial, sleep, psychosomatic, bowel control, motor/articulation, phobias, appetite and somatic) there were significant differences between the controls and the hearing impaired groups on only three. On two of these the hearing-impaired showed less disturbance in the areas of phobias and neuroticism. The third dimension combined a heterogeneous collection of features such as motor tics, verbal tics, enunciation, etc. It is therefore not surprising that the hearing-impaired group scored significantly higher on this dimension and for interpretation purposes it can be ignored.

When looking at peer relationships, the profoundly deaf especially, and to a lesser extent the partially hearing, appear to be at a disadvantage (see Table IV). The profoundly deaf subjects have significantly fewer peer contacts and are more teased and bullied than their hearing

Table III *The behaviour and temperament of deaf children—mean scores*

| | Groups | | | | Significance | |
	A = Controls	B = Residual speech retarded	C = Partially hearing	D = Profoundly deaf	A *vs* C	A *vs* D
Behaviour (parent interview)						
Global behaviour deviance						
(mean score)	42·9	43·1	39·9	39·2	NS	5%
Phobic dimension	6·1	6·4	4·8	5·5	1%	NS
Motor articulation dimension	2·9	5·3	4·06	4·90	1%	1%
Neurotic dimension	13·4	13·7	11·8	11·7	5%	5%
Temperament (parent interview)						
Mood	8·5	9·5	10·4	8·9	1%	NS
Irregularity	9·4	8·7	11·3	11·8	1%	1%

Table IV *Social relationships of deaf children*

	A = Controls	B = Partially hearing	C = Profoundly deaf	A *vs* B	A *vs* C
No. of peer contacts in last week	%	%	%		
9 or less	29	34	61		
10–29	51	47	21	NS	1%
30 or more	20	19	18		
Child bullied					
never	75	58	48	NS	1%
frequently occurs	25	42	52		
Child teased					
never in last year	62	37	32		
< 1 month	20	26	42	5%	1%
> 1 month	18	37	26		

counterparts. The partially hearing subjects are also significantly more teased than their normal hearing peers. Young children are inclined to be cruel, and therefore the present finding is not surprising; it suggests that hearing-impaired children are teased and bullied because of their handicap.

Temperament (Table III)

Of the four dimensions studied there were differences on only two. Both hearing impaired groups proved more irregular in temperament but only the partially hearing were significantly more moody than the controls.

Discussion and conclusions

At first glance our findings on behaviour appear contradictory in that teachers of the deaf report excess, and parents of the deaf report a relative lack of disturbed behaviour. However, in other major studies the agreement between teachers and parents about disturbance of behaviour has also been low (Rutter *et al.*, 1970a; Minde and Minde, 1977). In this case there are a number of possible explanations, but we will focus on three. First, the behaviour may be situation-specific and reveal itself only in the school setting where these deaf children are likely to be confronted with the realities of life; second, the parents may not be aware of the unusual nature of the behaviour; third, it may simply reflect the relative lack of exposure of parents to those pro-foundly deaf children who are in a residential school. We consider that the true explanation is likely to be a composite of all the three reasons given, the most important being the last of the three. In these circum-stances the most valid description of the children's behaviour is likely to be available from the school. Elsewhere we have pointed out that the mothers of the profoundly deaf appeared to be more resilient than the mothers of the partially hearing to the psychological stresses associated with coping with a handicapped child. In their review, Schlesinger and Meadow (1972) described contrasting research findings—some favour-ing residential students and others favouring day students. From such findings they go on to argue that there is likely to be an important interaction between school and family variables. Our findings tend to support this view, and we therefore agree with these authors that the issue of residential as against day schooling can only be evaluated meaningfully when all crucial factors are taken into consideration.

Turning to the teacher questionnaire, our data indicate that behavioural disturbance is related to the degree of hearing loss. However, a note of caution must be added. While the hearing of the profoundly deaf was significantly poorer than that of the partially hearing, transfer to a school for the profoundly deaf could occasionally have been influenced by social and behavioural criteria in the small number of marginal cases who could have easily fallen into either of the two deaf groups. Nevertheless, we do not consider that there are sufficient of these cases to produce differences of this magnitude; most of the differences are likely to be determined by the severity of deafness itself. These findings are not consistent with those of other workers such as Bowyer and Gillies (1972), but the studies are not really comparable as they have not used standardized tests covering the wide range of behaviours we have studied but rather a form of clinical impression consisting of judgement, by a variety of teachers, on two questions, namely, 'the ability to get on with other children' and 'the ability to get on with adults'. It is to be noted that the rate of psychiatric disturbance on the behaviour questionnaire we have used is from one and a half to three times as great as in the control group (see Table II) and therefore is broadly similar to Schlesinger and Meadow's (1972) findings using a teacher questionnaire. In addition our findings indicate that such disturbance more often than not tends to be of an antisocial variety.

When looking at peer relationships, the profoundly deaf especially, and to a lesser extent the partially hearing, appear to be worse off. The profoundly deaf subjects have significantly fewer peer contacts and are more teased and bullied than their hearing counterparts. The partially hearing subjects are also significantly more teased. Teasing and bullying by the hearing children seem to be important factors in accounting for the poorer peer relationships of the deaf. However, deafness itself must have played a part as it is entirely within expectation that certain children with communication difficulties will tend to be embarrassed by their poor speech, and also that poor speech itself will limit their ability to make satisfactory relationships.

The greater temperamental irregularity (patterns of eating and sleeping), may also stem from communication difficulties between the parents and their children. It could be argued that parents of the deaf have greater difficulties in communicating to their deaf children precisely what behaviour is expected of them at mealtimes or bedtimes, but these temperamental anomalies could also be explained by the previous finding that parents are more strict with them than with normal hearing children. It may simply be that they expect greater regularity or instantaneous obedience from them as ways of forestalling any dangers. The greater moodiness of the partially hearing may be a consequence of frustration caused by impatience with their difficulty in verbal communication. There is no simple plausible explanation of why moodiness is greater in the partially hearing than in the profoundly deaf group. On the other hand, impaired hearing is often associated with organic brain dysfunction and this might have contributed to the excess of moodiness and irregularity among the hearing-impaired children. However, our present findings provide no clues as to the relative contribution that communication difficulties and/or organic factors might have made to the behavioural problems displayed by the children.

Part III
Summary and Appendices

Summary

Background to the study

There have been few follow-up studies of children with delay of speech development which have attempted to assess outcome in a systematic and comprehensive manner. A unique opportunity for undertaking this type of longitudinal follow-up occurred as a result of the Newcastle Child Development Study (Neligan et al., 1974). In order to achieve this objective a series of preliminary simple steps were essential. First, we needed a definition of speech retardation: we decided to use the simple definition employed by the health visitors; this was the inability to use three or more words strung together to make some sort of sense by the age of 36 months. Second, it was necessary to select groups of children from a total population and to examine them at specified ages and by appropriate methods in order to identify the significant differences in their development. If such findings were to have wider validity it was essential for us to define the relationship between our study population and the total population from which it was drawn so that relevant comparisons could be made and conclusions drawn by workers located elsewhere.

The Newcastle Survey of Child Development enrolled survivors of the first month of life born in Newcastle during the years 1960–1962. This study gave us information, which had been collected by midwives, health visitors, doctors and teachers, about the children's first five years of life. This covered perinatal, obstetric and social data and also information about their health and development. Descriptions of the populations and other aspects of the study are provided in two previous publications (Neligan et al., 1974, 1976).

In order to broaden the study it was decided to include a hearing-impaired sample as this comprises a major group of children who, as a result of their deafness, suffer from varying degrees of speech retardation. It was impractical to limit the identification of hearing-impaired children of a narrow age group to the city of Newcastle upon Tyne alone, with its population of about a quarter of a million, as the prevalence of deafness is under two per 1000 children. Hence, in order to obtain a hearing-impaired sample which was statistically viable, it was necessary to recruit hearing-impaired children from the wider Tyneside area complex. This was facilitated by the co-operation of the regional child otologist.

As our aim is to provide the reader with a brief résumé of the contents of the book we have included in the summary only major themes, findings and related conclusions. Inevitably, therefore, some important themes will be found only on perusal of the full text.

1 Speech retarded children

Aims and objectives of study

The aim of the study was to obtain a comprehensive picture of the intellectual, behavioural and physical functioning of children at school age who had an early history of speech retardation. At this stage of their development a wide range of reliable and valid assessments could be undertaken. The method described above would obviate the pitfalls associated with retrospective studies and the use of biased samples recruited from specialist clinics or hospitals. Further, we wished to study a total population of speech retarded children in a way and at a depth which we do not believe has been previously achieved by any other group of workers. It was also our intention to undertake a clinical and statistical classification of the children involved and to estimate the prevalence of their handicaps.

Method

The progress of the children with speech delay was compared with that of a matched control group. The latter consisted of children who did not suffer from speech delay and who were matched individually with our study cases on three criteria—sex, age and family neighbourhood. However, in the comparisons between the subgroups and the controls matching was not maintained—the total control group was used for every comparison. This control group was also used for comparison with the hearing impaired sample.

The groups of children were compared on a variety of measures: speech and language, intelligence, educational achievement, behavioural and neurological assessment. We were also able to relate early social, family and medical factors to current functioning.

Of the 3300 children born in Newcastle upon Tyne in 1962, 133, which constitutes 4% of the population, were identified as speech retarded. Of these, 102 were studied more intensively when they were seven to eight years old.

Losses

The remaining 31 cases of the original 133 were not available for comprehensive study at school age: two had died; 21 cases had left the area; eight cases had to be excluded from detailed analysis because of insufficient data (see Chapter 1). However, the information available on the 29 surviving children showed that the rate of serious handicaps in this group was no greater than that of the group of children available for assessment; in addition, the distribution of occupational social class of their families tended to be slightly better than those who we were able to study. We therefore concluded that those not seen were likely to be broadly similar to those who were assessed. An appropriate adjustment has been made for these losses when estimating prevalence.

Diagnosis and classification

A summary profile of the performance of the various groups (with the exception of the pathological deviant group) of children at age seven or eight is presented in Table I. This table shows the differences between the groups on a large number of measures of intelligence, language, speech and educational and behavioural performance. Furthermore, as the children were assessed clincially at the age of seven years our diagnostic assessment allowed us to classify speech retarded children into two broad subgroups, which we have labelled *pathological deviant* and *residual speech retarded*. The pathological deviant group consisted of children whose functioning intellectually, psychologically or physically was indubitably abnormal. It included children with severe disorders of communication (autism, elective mutism, dysphasia and dysarthria) and intellectual-cum-physical handicaps (cerebral palsy and subnormality). Some 18 (17·6%) of the 102 cases studied fell into the pathological deviant category. The Residual Speech Retarded Group comprised the remaining children. They displayed no obvious serious handicap on clinical assessment at the age of seven years.

A further clinical classification was undertaken. This was dependent on whether these children suffered from *speech retardation alone* or whether they suffered from *retardation of both speech and walking*. In short, we identified three subgroups: those who walked early comprised the specific speech delayed group; those who walked late comprised the

Table I *Summary of findings comparing control and study groups*

	Normal control group	Specific speech delayed group	Intermediate delayed group	General delayed group	Partial hearing group	Profoundly deaf group
Full-scale IQ (WISC)	—	—	—	—	—	X
Non-verbal tests:						
Perceptual quotient (Frostig)	—	O	—	—	—	—
Conceptual maturity (Harris' D-A-M)	O	O	—	—	—	—
Manual dexterity (Purdue pegboard)	O	O	—	—	X	X
Memory cards (Skemp)	O	—	—	—	X	X
Paired associates (Skemp)	O	—	—	—	X	X
Visual concepts (Skemp)	O	—	—	—	X	X
Auditory visual integration (Birch)	O	—	—	—	X	X
Haptic-visual integration (Birch)	O	O	O	O	X	X
Imitation of gestures	O	—	—	—	X	X
Picture completion (WISC)	O	O	O	O	O	—
Picture arrangement (WISC)	—	—	—	—	O	—
Block design (WISC)	O	—	—	—	O	—
Object assembly (WISC)	O	O	O	O	O	O
Coding (WISC)	O	O	—	—	O	O
Performance IQ (WISC)	O	O	—	—	O	—
Visual association (ITPA)	O	—	—	—	O	—
Visual closure (ITPA)	O	—	—	—	O	—
Manual expression (ITPA)	O	—	—	—	O	+
Visual sequential memory (ITPA)	O	—	—	—	O	—
Visual reception (ITPA)	O	O	—	—	—	—
Verbal and language tests:						
Information (WISC)	—	—	—	—	—	X
Comprehension (WISC)	O	O	—	—	—	X
Arithmetic (WISC)	O	—	—	—	—	X
Similarities (WISC)	—	—	—	—	—	X
Vocabulary (WISC)	—	—	—	—	—	X
Verbal IQ (WISC)	—	—	—	—	—	X

	Normal control group	*Specific speech delayed group*	*Intermediate delayed group*	*General delayed group*	*Partial hearing group*	*Profoundly deaf group*
Verbal expression (ITPA)	—	—	—	—	—	X
Grammatic closure (ITPA)	—	—	—	—	—	X
Auditory association (ITPA)	—	—	—	—	—	X
Auditory sequential memory (ITPA)	—	—	—	—	—	X
Auditory reception (ITPA)	O	—	—	—	—	X
Language quotient (ITPA)	—	—	—	—	X	X
Sound blending (ITPA)	—	—	—	—	X	X
Auditory closure (ITPA)	—	—	—	—	X	X
Vocabulary comprehension (EPVT)	—	—	—	—	X	X
Simple sentence	+	+	—	—	X	X
Simple-plus sentence	O	O	O	O	X	X
Compound sentence	O	O	O	O	X	X
Complex sentence	O	—	—	—	X	X
Sentence complexity (Global score)	O	O	—	—	X	X
Mean sentence length (Bus story)	—	—	—	—	X	X
Information content score	—	—	—	—	X	X
Incomplete sentences (Bus story)	O	—	—	—	X	X
Reading quotient (Schonell)	—	—	—	—	O	—
Speech						
Immature articulation score	—	—		O	X	X
Correct articulation score	—	—		O	X	X
Behaviour/personality						
Behaviour adjustment (Rutter scale B: Total score)	O	O	—		O	—
Antisocial score (Rutter scale B)	O	O	O	O	O	—
Neurotic subscore (Rutter scale B)	O	O	O	O	O	O
Extraversion (JEPI)	O	—	—		X	X
Neuroticism (JEPI)	O	O	O	O	X	X
Lie scale (JEPI)	O	O	O	O	X	X

+ significantly better than controls
O no significant difference from controls
— significantly poorer than controls
X no data available because test not administered

general delayed group; and those whose walking milestones were average comprised the intermediate group. Such simple subcategorizations have served to underline the heterogeneity of problems which are likely to be found amongst children who were previously speech retarded.

The value of a simple speech screen at the age of three years

The predictive value of this simple screen is fully described in Chapter 1. Of the 4% of children in the population identified as speech retarded, one in five was later found to be suffering from some serious language and intellectual or physical handicap and these constitute the pathological deviant subgroup. We initially thought that the remaining children (the Residual Speech Retarded Group) could be considered as falling into the so-called developmental speech disorder category. However, this proved to be mainly true of the children found to be suffering from specific speech delay.

Prevalence—incidence of disorders

As many of the conditions which we have studied were very rare and indeed only manifested in one or two cases in our sample, our conclusions regarding the prevalence of those conditions must be very tentative.

It has also been pointed out that precise figures for the number of children with speech and language disorders are difficult to obtain and that more data are needed. Our data, which were epidemiologically based, may contribute to a more accurate estimate of the incidence of some of the language disorders. As we were unable to interview about 25% of the children identified by our screen we have corrected our estimates by multiplying our speech disorder rates by a factor of 1·30.

We found that retardation of speech among three-year-olds is a relatively common problem which affects 4% of the population of Newcastle upon Tyne. Such a figure is broadly in agreement with the earlier findings of Morley (1965) in the same region of England, and with the national figures quoted for the USA by Marge (1972). We also report a crude prevalence rate of 0·8 per 1000 children for autism which is consistent with the findings from other studies (Lotter, 1966) but a prevalence of 0·4 per 1000 children for elective mutism and severe childhood dysphasia respectively, which suggests that the two latter conditions are as rare as, or perhaps even rarer than, infantile autism. The rarity of these conditions may well explain the absence of detailed information about their features and aetiology.

Influence of socio-cultural factors

We had attempted to control occupational social class differences between the groups by matching each speech retarded child with another child of the same age and sex and from the same neighbourhood. However, when sociological factors were studied in depth it was found there was an excess of adverse socio-cultural indices in the case of the Residual Speech Retarded Group as compared with the control group. Our attempts therefore to control for social class and environmental factors were only partially successful. We therefore concluded that even within the same urban area or neighbourhood there was a relationship between child handicap and adverse social factors. In addition, the mothers of the Residual Speech Retarded Group had high rates of serious psychological problems. After a careful examination of the relationships and relevant issues we further concluded that these were more likely to be a reflection of tensions associated with the greater loadings of adverse social factors already described. We were surprised by the low rates of serious disturbance reported by the mothers of the pathological deviant group. We speculate that special facilities for care of these children and opportunities for working may have protective or modifying influences.

Quantitative assessment of mother's speech was also undertaken and no differences were found between groups on a variety of measures. In a study of speech disorders of childhood it is important to ascertain whether there is any evidence of a family history of similar problems. We identified an excess of such problems in the case of the parents of the Residual Speech Retarded Group and we consider that this confirms the aetiological importance of such factors. Such evidence gives rise to the hypothesis that there is a developmental component with a familial basis in at least a subgroup of the Residual Speech Retarded Group.

Predictive importance of speech delay

Compared with their normal peers (that is with the control group), the Residual Speech Retarded Group was shown to have varying degrees of impairment in the areas of speech, language, intellectual and educational functioning and also to be more poorly adjusted in behaviour. These differences cannot be attributed solely to differences in social environment because we had controlled as far as possible by matching for such factors; hence while the Residual Speech Retarded Group had a slight downward gradient of occupational social class this was not at all statistically significant.

However, the more sensitive measure of social environment, which we have labelled the social risk index, did show significant differences between the groups. It was therefore necessary to determine whether such a factor made any important independent contribution to the poor performance of the Residual Speech Retarded Group as compared to the controls. We checked this by means of a partialling out technique in relation to 13 measures of performance and found that when we made allowance for the influence of social factors as represented by the social risk index, the picture for practical purposes remained largely unchanged in the case of the total Residual Speech Retarded Group, and virtually unchanged in the case of the specific speech delayed subgroup in comparison with the control group. We therefore concluded that differences in social environment between the speech and control groups were not sufficient to significantly affect outcome.

The results of the cognitive tests are best summarized by study of the principal component analysis. Here we found that the cognitive functioning of the Residual Speech Retarded Group differed significantly from the control group on the first two components. On the first component, which we termed 'general cognitive ability' the Residual Speech Retarded Group obtained an inferior score and hence as a group has a poorer level of general intellectual ability. On the second component, a bipolar one which we termed 'perceptual-motor ability' versus 'verbal ability', the Residual Speech Retarded Group differed from the control in that the mean scores of the former group tended towards the 'perceptual-motor' pole of the bipolar component and away from the 'verbal ability pole'. We conclude, therefore, that as a group, the Residual Speech Retarded children not only had a comparatively lower level of general intellectual ability but their tendency was to rely more heavily on visuo-motor skills rather than verbal-symbolic skills. Such differences in performance between the Residual Speech Retarded Group and the control group are consistent with expectations and underline important differences between their cognitive style.

Various tests of those subgroups identified on the basis of their speech and walking milestones showed that they differed from the controls in some important respects. The intellectual performance of the specific speech delayed group (i.e. those who walked early) was broadly similar to that described as being characteristic of children considered to be dysphasic (Olson, 1961; Weiner, 1972). These findings therefore provide circumstantial evidence that our group of children with a specific delay in speech had previously suffered from a type of developmental dysphasia. Other circumstantial evidence in support of this hypothesis is as follows: children in the specific speech delayed group were found to have a good non-verbal IQ in contrast to their relatively poor grammatical abilities, vocabulary, comprehension and expression of ideas and poor reading attainment, poor word sound (phoneme) discrimination and immaturity of articulation of speech. On the other hand, the occupational social class of the breadwinners did not significantly differ from that of the breadwinners of their normal peers and the hearing of these children was within normal limits. Our specific speech delayed group therefore appears to represent the less severe end of the spectrum of the developmental language disorder syndrome described by Ingram (1972) in which the prognosis is considered to be reasonably good. In contrast, the children in the general delayed group were found to be grossly retarded in their language, verbal and non-verbal intelligence and educational attainments, but not significantly so in speech articulation.

Our findings also emphasize the important relationship between earlier retardation of speech and subsequent impairment in reading, although this is not a new finding (Ingram, 1972). Furthermore, both subgroups of speech retarded children showed impaired ability to discriminate between units of word sounds. We therefore postulate that such defects may constitute one of the important basic mechanisms underlying the reading difficulties of these groups.

The finding that a high percentage of residual speech retarded children display significant impairment of intelligence, language and educational achievement is of major importance to clinicians, educationalists and parents. It implies that children who had speech delay in early childhood are likely to require careful assessment and appropriate remedial action at school age or even earlier. In addition, the prognosis in terms of disturbed behaviour is likewise poor but particularly so in the case of those children with more severe degrees of speech disorders. The pattern that has been found is that of introversion and withdrawal, and is, with some exceptions, similar to that often described in the literature as characteristic of children with speech and language disorders.

Multivariate analyses

The main aim of the multivariate analyses was to investigate the inter-correlations of some of the basic data on our group of residual speech retarded children. The first technique used for this purpose was McQuitty's (1957) technique of cluster analysis: here one main cluster was identified which we labelled a cognitive cluster. The cluster illustrates the considerable importance of a subsequent comprehension deficit in children who were previously speech retarded. The most important finding of this cluster analysis is the central and pivotal nature of the measure of vocabulary comprehension (the English Picture Vocabulary Test) which correlates significantly, though not necessarily highly, with the majority of the remaining variables. There is in addition a subcluster which includes the variable language literacy index of the mother; this is mainly associated with a fairly high level of immature errors of articulation in the child. Various explanations are offered for this correlation.

Factorial analysis was undertaken on data based on the Residual Speech Retarded Group. Our findings indicate a contrast between, on the one hand, good verbal abilities of the child (articulation, vocabulary and grammar), good language ability of mother and positive social environmental influences, and on the other hand, uneven physical maturation associated with relatively good non-verbal intellectual abilities (see Chapter 7). These and other findings lead us to two conclusions. First, that social and environmental stimulation may be important facilitators of the development of speech, language and verbal abilities. Second, that poor early speech development accompanied by satisfactory motor milestone development does not necessarily give rise to a poor intellectual outcome. This is particularly true of practical abilities. Furthermore, the findings described above also constitute support for the notion of a specific developmental speech/language disorder syndrome.

Sex differences

The male:female ratio for our total speech retarded group was 1·7:1. When the Residual Speech Retarded Group and the pathologically deviant group were analysed separately, the male:female ratio was 2:1 for the former and 1:1 for the latter. The former is in broad agreement with the findings in most of developmental disorders where male:female ratios are in the order of 2:1 to 3:1.

2 Hearing-impaired children

In collaboration with the University-based child otologist who provided a regional reference service for Tyneside, a total of 59 hearing-impaired children were identified. The control group used in the study of speech retarded children were again used as controls for our study of hearing-impaired children. As the children in the hearing-impaired group were a year older than those in the control group comparisons had to be made with caution. However, age-corrected tests were usually employed, which in the circumstances, allow as far as is possible valid comparisons.

Diagnosis and classification

As with the speech retarded group, clinical assessments were undertaken in order to identify a pathologically deviant group of children.

(a) *Pathologically deviant hearing-impaired group* This was a smaller group than anticipated, consisting of one severely subnormal child, three brain-damaged or spastic children and one with a cleft palate.

(b) *Hearing-impaired children without significant organic impairment* This group comprised the remaining 54 children who were functioning sufficiently well in their school settings to be able to respond readily to testing. These children were divided into two subgroups: the partially hearing (21 cases) and the profoundly deaf (33 cases). We confine our discussion to the above 54 cases.

Social and family background

The occupational social class of the parents of the hearing-impaired group did not significantly differ from the control group, nor was there any significant excess of other indices of social and family pathology.

In contrast, comparison of the hearing-impaired and control groups with regard to difficulty in early development revealed a somewhat complicated picture. The hearing-impaired group had suffered from more than the usual number of minor fevers (measles, mumps, etc.) and also major infections (meningitis/encephalitis). On the other hand, of the two subgroups of hearing-impaired children, the profoundly deaf group had suffered significantly more postnatal illness than the partially hearing group and also a significant excess of epileptic fits compared with the control group. In profoundly deaf children such illnesses were more likely to occur in the first five years of life.

Some of the more striking findings related to the attitudes and psychological reactions of parents of deaf children. Despite the apparent stress of having a child with severe deafness, mothers of profoundly deaf children were found to have a lower incidence of treatment of 'nervousness' than mothers of normal hearing children; in contrast, the highest incidence of 'nervousness' was noted in mothers of partially hearing children. As most of the profoundly deaf children attended residential schools, and the majority of partially hearing did not, we suggest that the mothers of the profoundly deaf did not have as much in the way of daily stresses associated with attending to a handicapped child, and this may be the basis of their lower levels of 'nervousness'. Such a finding may constitute an argument in favour of residential schooling.

We can summarize the salient differences of parental attitudes as follows: in the case of the hearing-impaired group the mother more usually than the father assumed the disciplinary role, whereas in the case of the control group it was usually the father who did so. Furthermore, despite the greater strictness and supervision shown by the parents of the hearing-impaired group towards their handicapped child, these parents had fewer expectations of their child than had those of the control group, and this was particularly evident in the case of the profoundly deaf group. Our findings suggest a greater degree of over-protection in the parents of the hearing-impaired children. Such attitudinal differences may be important determinants of the slower social maturation of hearing-impaired children compared with normal hearing children which is often reported in the literature (Myklebust, 1964).

The amount of communication between parents and their deaf children appeared to be related to the severity of their deafness. In addition, there were differences in the type of communication in that the parents of the profoundly deaf children were more inclined to use baby talk with their children.

Non-verbal cognitive abilities

The non-verbal cognitive attainments of the hearing-impaired group were found to be significantly poorer than those of the normal control group. Moreover, the mean scores of the hearing-impaired group were usually nearer to those of the Residual Speech Retarded Group than to those of the control group. These results were consistent for a variety of such cognitive tests, namely, the Draw-a-Man Test of conceptual maturity, the Frostig Developmental Test of Visual Perception, the non-verbal subtests of the Illinois Test of Psycholinguistic Ability and the performance subtests of the Wechster Intelligence Scale for Children. This trend of differences between the three groups was also found on the principal component analysis with regard to the first component, which measured non-verbal intelligence: the hearing-impaired did worst, the controls best and the Residual Speech Retarded Group obtained an intermediate score.

It is argued that it would be an oversimplification, if not erroneous, to conclude that the hearing-impaired are 'less intelligent' than their hearing counterparts. It is more useful to consider the findings on the second component of the principal component analysis. On this bipolar component of 'visual symbolic ability' versus 'motor ability' the mean score of the hearing-impaired group falls at the 'motor pole', that of the controls at the 'visual symbolic pole' and that of the Residual Speech Retarded Group in between. This suggests that there are differences in cognitive style between the groups of children studied.

Subclassification of hearing-impaired group and profile of abilities

The division of the hearing-impaired group into profoundly deaf and partially hearing subgroups according to whether they attended a school for the profoundly deaf or a school for the partially hearing highlighted the importance of distinguishing between children with differences in severity of hearing loss, albeit on the basis of a simple classification.

Compared to the normal control group the profoundly deaf group almost always scored significantly worse on the cognitive tests used while the partially hearing group did not. On one subtest alone (manual expression) the profoundly deaf group did score significantly better than the other three groups. In contrast, on the majority of non-verbal tasks the performance of the partially hearing in many ways resembled that of the normal control group and in some cases proved to be better than that of the Residual Speech Retarded Group.

Compared with those of the control, the Residual Speech Retarded and the partially hearing groups, the test performances of the pro-foundly deaf were in general worse (and almost always significantly so when compared to the control group). A characteristic of the profoundly deaf group was the patchiness of their subtest scores. This was clearly highlighted on the ITPA (visuo-motor tests only) where the profoundly deaf group obtained a superior subtest score over the other three groups on a test of manual expression. It would seem that where the mode of language used is more concrete—in that it involved manual gesture—and meaningful to the child then hearing loss is no impediment. Nevertheless, our findings suggest that, in the main, severity of hearing loss is an important factor which contributes to the poorer intellectual and educa-tional performance of hearing-impaired children.

The partially hearing group showed a clear trend of superiority over their profoundly deaf counterparts, and in some instances did even better than the Residual Speech Retarded Group. In short, the partially hearing in many ways resembled the normal control group.

Behaviour and personality

Some of the findings based on two different sources of information at first sight appear contradictory. While the parents of the hearing-impaired group report less in the way of neurotic and antisocial behaviour compared with the control group, teachers report more. Possible explana-tions for these differences are discussed in Chapter 11. There are two other important findings: the first is that the profoundly deaf children display more serious maladjustment (on the Rutter teacher's scale) than the control and the partially hearing children; hence, severity of maladjustment in school appears to be related to degree of deafness. The second is that the main type of maladjustment shown by the profoundly deaf in school is of an antisocial rather than a neurotic variety.

On the basis of parents' reports, it is mainly in terms of social maladjustment that the hearing-impaired group show excesses compared with the control group. Again, it is the profoundly deaf group who show the poorest adjustment. Finally, significantly greater degrees of irregularity are reported for both the hearing-impaired groups, and a significantly greater degree of moodiness for the partially hearing group alone.

We offer the tentative explanation that the partially hearing group is inclined to vent their psychological frustrations in moodiness whereas the profoundly deaf are likely to resort to antisocial behaviour. Other possible psychological and organic explanations are offered in Chapter 11. It is evident that the behaviour of the hearing-impaired children tends to be situation-specific.

Appendix 1
Supplementary tables

Part I—The speech retarded study

Chapter 1

Table 1   *Schooling*

Special placements	Total =	19
(a) ESN schools		8
(b) Spastic schools		1
(c) Deaf schools		2
(d) Training centre		3
(e) Subnormality hospitals		2
(f) Not at school—ineducable		3
Ordinary schools	Total =	83
	Grand total	102

Chapter 3

Table 2   *Psychological tests*

		Controls	Residual speech retarded	*Significance*
WISC full scale IQ	m	96·26	88·3	c
	s.d.	9·9	10·96	
WISC verbal IQ	m	92·5	84·3	c
	s.d.	9·97	9·19	

(cont.)

Table 2 (*cont.*)

		Controls	Residual speech retarded	*Significance*
WISC performance IQ	m	101·17	94·94	[b]
	s.d.	11·04	13·27	
WISC V/P discrepancy	m	8·69	10·41	NS
	s.d.	10·75	10·77	
Frostig (motor perceptual quotient)	m	95·99	86·82	[c]
	s.d.	11·91	14·07	
Harris DAM (conceptual maturity)	m	96·35	92·4	[b]
	s.d.	9·93	9·11	
Skemp (visual concept formation)	m	23·52	21·83	[b]
	s.d.	1·53	2·44	
Birch (auditory visual integration)	m	6·23	5·02	[b]
	s.d.	2·8	2·03	
Purdue Pegboard (manual dexterity)	m	8·64	8·1	[b]
	s.d.	1·29	1·48	
Imitation of gesture[a]	m	30·86	34·10	[c]
	s.d.	5·60	6·65	

[a] The lower the score, the better the performance, the higher the score, the poorer the performance.
[b] $p < 0.01$ [c] $p < 0.001$ NS = not significant

Table 2A *Educational attainment*

		Controls	Residual speech retarded	Significance
Reading quotient (Schonell)	m	93·94	80·38	[c]
	s.d.	19·15	15·68	

Table 3   *Distribution of WISC scores*

	WISC full scale		scale IQ		Performance IQ	
	Controls					
	a		b		c	
	n	%	n	%	n	%
116 or more	4	4	2	2	12	12
101–115	35	35	24	24	44	44
86–100	49	49	53	53	37	37
71–85	12	12	21	21	7	7
70 or less	0		0		0	0
Total		100		100		100

	WISC full scale IQ		Verbal IQ		Performance IQ	
			Residual speech retarded			
	d		e		f	
	n	%	n	%	n	%
116 or more	1	1·25	0	0	6	7·34
101–115	11	13·75	7	8·75	25	30·48
86–100	37	46·25	30	37·50	34	41·46
71–85	26	32·50	37	46·25	16	19·51
70 or less	5	6·25	6	7·50	1	1·21
Total	80		80		82	

Note Appropriate cells have been collapsed to produce 2 × 4 table for chi-squared with 3 d.f.

a *vs* d $\chi^2 = 24$ $p < 0.001$
b *vs* e $\chi^2 = 23$ $p < 0.001$
c *vs* f $\chi^2 = 9.8$ $p < 0.01$

Table 4   *Speech and language measures*

Measure	Controls[a] ($n = 101$)		Residual speech retarded ($n = 80$)		Significance
	m	s.d.	m	s.d.	*t* test
1 *ITPA*					
Psycholinguistic quotient	91·3	10·1	80·9	10·2	c
Representational level— scaled score	32·7	3·6	29·1	4·0	b
Automatic level— scaled score	33/8	6·0	30·8	6·2	c
Psycholinguistic age (months)	81·5	5·1	73·2	9·1	c
2 *Sentence analysis*					
Mean words per sentence	13·2	2·4	11·2	2·6	c
Sentence complexity	36·7	7·2	32·6	9·7	b
Content score	30·0	6·2	25·3	7·9	b
Incomplete sentences	0·38	0·69	0·9	1·6	b
3 *EPVT*	94	10·8	81·2	11·6	c

(*cont.*)

Table 4 (*cont.*)

Measure	Controls[a] (n = 101)	Residual speech retarded (n = 80)	Significance
4 *Communication style* (follows Bernstein)	Absolute nos	Absolute nos	Chi-squared
Grade (i) Highly elaborated	7	3	$\chi^2 = 14.5$
(ii) Elaborated	35	13	d.f. = 2
(iii) Moderate	43	35	
(iv) Restricted	16	26	c
(v) Highly restricted	0	3	

[a] For some tests n = 100
[b] $p < 0.01$ [c] $p < 0.001$

Table 5   *Assessment of speech at seven years using Edinburgh articulation test*

		Controls (n = 100)	Residual speech retarded (n = 80)	Statistical difference
Correct score	m	59.5	52.5	
	s.d.	8.6	12.4	$p < 0.01$
Immature errors of articulation	m	4.9	9.9	
	s.d.	6.2	7.6	$p < 0.01$

Table 6   *Distribution of immature errors of articulation*

Range	Controls	Residual speech retarded	
0–5	65	24	(30%)
6–14	26	40	(50%)
15+	9	16	(20%)

Sig. $\chi^2 = 21.9$, 2 d.f., $p < 0.01$

Table 7   *Principal component analysis—controls plus Residual Speech Retarded Group*

Variable	Factor I variance 33·8% general Weight[a]	II 4·9% bipolar Weight
ITPA auditory association	0·82	0·26
ITPA grammatic closure	0·82	0·23
EPVT (vocabulary comprehension)	0·79	0·10
Bus story information	0·76	0·15
ITPA auditory closure	0·75	0·22
WISC vocabulary	0·75	0·25
WISC picture arrangement	0·72	−0·00
ITPA verbal expression	0·72	0·10
Schonell reading	0·72	0·23
Bus story sentence length	0·71	0·22
ITPA visual closure	0·67	−0·27
WISC information	0·66	0·19
Frostig spatial rel.	0·66	−0·36
figure ground	0·61	−0·38
ITPA auditory seq. memory	0·65	0·17
ITPA auditory reception	0·65	0·18
Harris DAM	0·59	−0·30
Integration auditory/visual	0·58	0·06
Bus story complex sentence	0·63	0·25
Skemp visual concepts	0·60	−0·12
WISC arithmetic	0·62	0·15
WISC object assembly	0·53	−0·44
WISC picture completion	0·45	−0·39
WISC block design	0·58	−0·37
Integration haptic/visual	0·21	−0·36
Purdue—manual dexterity	0·55	−0·35
ITPA sound blending	0·55	0·30
WISC similarities	0·41	0·26
Intepretation	General cognitive ability	Perceptual motor organization *vs* verbal ability

[a] For convenience only the highest weights have been included thereby reducing the number of variables from 44 to 28

Table 8   *Principal component analysis: group comparison*

	Controls (n = 100)		Residual speech retarded (n = 80)		Significance
	m	s.d.	m	s.d.	
Component I (general cognitive ability)	1·6271	3·175	−1·9751	3·7013	p <0·001
Component II (verbal ability *vs* perceptual-motor organization)	0·2154	1·362	−0·2681	1·587	p <0·02

Chapter 4

Table 9   *Psychiatric disorder rated by psychologist*

Severity	a = Controls	b = Residual Speech Retarded Group	c = pathological speech retarded group	Significance 5%	1%
Nil	92	58	1		
Some	9	21	3	a *vs* b a *vs* c b *vs* c	
Marked	0	3	14		
Other	1	2	0		

Table 10   *Psychological assessment—child's attitude*

Feature	Degree	a = Controls	b = RSRG	Significance 5%	1%
Level of confidence of child	high	89	55		
	moderate	12	26	a *vs* b	
	poor	0	1		
Attention span of child	good	63	30		
	moderate	35	44	a *vs* b	
	poor	1	8		

Table 11   *Correlation analyses—behaviour, intelligence and language*

	Controls	Residual Speech Retarded Group
IQ and LQ	0·74[c]	0·83[c]
IQ and behaviour	−0·30[b]	−0·26[a]
LQ and behaviour	−0·41[b]	−0·35[b]
n =	100	80

[a] p <0·05
[b] p <0·01
[c] p <0·001

LQ = Language quotient on ITPA;IQ = Verbal intelligence on WISC; Behaviour = Rutter 'B' Scale total score.

Traditionally, good intelligence is denoted by a high score on an IQ test but good behaviour is denoted by a low score. Hence if children with high IQs tend to have good behaviour and children with low IQs poor behaviour, then a negative correlation can be expected.

Chapter 5

Table 12 *Comparison of means of controls and of the three subgroups of speech retarded children—cognition and language*

Measures		a = Controls (n = 100)	b = Early walkers (specific delay) (n = 24)	c = Int. walkers (intermediate group) (n = 31)	d = Late walkers (general delay) (n = 22)	Significance 5%	1%	0.1%
Cognitive								
Frostig (Vis. Percept.)	m	95·9	86·8	90·9	78·8	b vs d	c vs d	a vs d, a vs b
DAM (Draw-a-Man)	m	96·4	94·9	92·6	87·3	c vs d	b vs d	a vs d
EPVT (Eng. Pic. Vocab)	m	94·0	84·6	82·4	76·5	—	b vs d, a vs b	a vs d
Prudue (Manual Dex.)	m	8·6	8·5	8·1	7·6	b vs d, a vs c	a vs d	a vs c
Birch A/V integration	m	6·2	5·1	5·0	4·9	a vs d, a vs c	—	—
Birch H/V integration	m	7·5	7·5	7·4	7·1	—	—	—
Skemp memory concepts	m	7·7	7·7	6·9	6·2	—	a vs d, b vs d	a vs c
Skemp paired association	m	18·6	18·6	16·6	16·0	—	b vs d, a vs c, a vs d	—
Skemp visual concepts	m	23·5	22·9	22·0	20·7	b vs d	—	a vs c, a vs d
Imitation of gestures[a]	m	30·9	32·7	34·6	35·9	—	—	a vs c, a vs d
Full scale IQ (WISC)	m	96·3	91·2	88·5	83·3	a vs b, b vs d	—	a vs c, a vs d
Performance IQ	m	101·2	98·9	97·7	88·6	b vs d	—	a vs d
Verbal IQ	m	92·5	85·4	84·8	81·2	—	a vs b	a vs d

		a	b	c	d			
Reading quotient (Schonell)	m	93·9	82·5	81·0	76·2	—	a vs b	a vs c / a vs d
Language quotient (ITPA)	m	91·3	84·1	82·2	76·2	—	a vs b	a vs c / a vs d
Syntax								
Sentence complexity (global score)	m	36·7	33·7	33·8	30·9	—	a vs d	—
Frequency of use of different types of sentence complexity								
simple	m	4·15	5·41	5·32	4·77	a vs b / a vs c	—	—
simple-plus	m	2·67	2·91	3·03	3·23	—	—	—
compound	m	1·58	1·29	1·52	1·41	—	—	—
complex	m	5·62	4·70	4·58	3·72	a vs c	a vs d	a vs d
Information content	m	30·0	26·8	25·8	23·7	a vs b	a vs c	a vs c
Mean sentence length	m	13·2	11·4	11·4	10·7	—	a vs b	a vs d
Incomplete sentences[a]	m	0·4	0·8	0·9	1·1	—	a vs c / a vs d	—
Speech								
Correct articulation	m	58·5	54·3	52·0	56·6	a vs b	—	a vs c
Immature errors[a]	m	4·9	9·8	10·5	7·6	a vs b	a vs c	—
WISC verbal/performance discrepancy (mean of P minus V IQ)	m	8·7	13·2	9·6	7·5	a vs b	—	—

[a] The lower the score the better the performance; the higher the score the poorer the performance. On all other variables the higher the score the better the performance.

Owing to volume of data the standard deviations have been excluded.

Table 13   *ITPA subtest scaled scores of normal controls, specific speech delayed, intermediate and general delayed groups*

Subtest	a = Controls (n = 101)	b = Specific speech delayed (n = 24)	c = Intermediate (n = 31)	d = General delayed (n = 22)	Significance 5%	Significance 1%	Significance 0·1%
	m	m	m	m			
Auditory reception	33·14	30·20	29·90	27·73	a *vs* c	—	a *vs* d
Visual reception	28·87	28·75	27·61	24·36	—	—	a *vs* d
Auditory association	33·80	28·33	26·87	25·55	—	a *vs* b	a *vs* c a *vs* d
Visual association	31·11	29·71	28·39	26·46	a *vs* c	a *vs* d	—
Verbal expression	36·94	34·79	34·07	32·73	a *vs* c	a *vs* b	a *vs* c
Manual expression	32·80	31·71	31·07	29·27	a *vs* c	—	a *vs* d
Grammatic closure	36·80	29·42	29·35	25·77	—	—	a *vs* b a *vs* c
Visual closure	30·11	29·25	27·16	24·05	a *vs* c	—	a *vs* d
Auditory sequential memory	34·14	29·83	30·42	28·46	—	a *vs* b a *vs* c	a *vs* d
Visual sequential memory	33·80	31·83	31·26	29·10	a *vs* c	a *vs* d	—
Supplementary subtest							
Auditory closure	25·38	18·12	19·45	18·04	—	—	a *vs* b a *vs* c
Sound blending	47·14	43·70	44·03	43·41	—	—	a *vs* b a *vs* c

Table 14 WISC subtest scaled scores of normal controls, specific speech delayed, intermediate and general delayed groups

Subtest	a = Controls (n = 100)	b = Specific speech delayed (n = 24)	c = Intermediate (n = 31)	d = General delayed (n = 22)	Significance 5%	Significance 1%	Significance 0.1%
	m	m	m	m			
Information	8·65	6·54	7·29	6·36	—	a vs c	a vs b a vs d
Comprehension	7·19	6·96	6·42	6·04	—	a vs d	—
Arithmetic	10·22	9·67	9·10	8·14	b vs d a vs c	a vs d	—
Similarities	8·94	7·54	7·55	7·45	—	a vs d	—
Vocabulary	9·05	7·50	7·58	7·18	—	a vs b a vs c a vs d	a vs b a vs c a vs d
Picture completion	10·80	11·75	9·87	9·86	b vs d	—	—
Picture arrangement	9·37	8·33	8·29	7·45	a vs b a vs c	—	—
Block design	10·50	10·00	9·39	8·50	b vs d a vs c	a vs d	—
Object assembly	10·33	9·54	9·58	9·04	—	—	—
Coding	9·79	9·17	9·10	6·95	b vs d	—	a vs d

Chapter 6

Table 15 *Correlation matrix—data included in first principal component analysis*

Variables	1	2	3	4	5	6	7	8	9	10	11	12
1 Social class												
2 Sex	00											
3 EPVT	-29[b]	34[b]										
4 A–V integration	-30[b]	-02	33[b]									
5 Communication code	35[b]	-02	-42[b]	-42[b]								
6 Right/left differences	09	03	-19	-20	13							
7 Imitation of gestures	07	07	-25[a]	-20	32[b]	20						
8 Immature errors of articulation	15	16	-05	-14	18	-03	11					
9 Hearing impairment	25[a]	-26[a]	-26[b]	-15	14	12	-03	03				
10 Scatter WISC	-16	21	32[b]	23[a]	-22[a]	-16	-20	-16	-06			
11 Scatter ITPA	-12	-13	-17	00	-14	-07	00	-02	17	09		
12 General milestone delay	00	-01	-27[b]	-07	09	32[b]	19	02	-04	-20	16	
13 Language literacy index mother	24[a]	11	-08	-23[a]	08	-03	-18	28[b]	06	20	08	07

[a] Significant at 5%   [b] Significant at 1%
Error scores—variables 1,5,6,7,8,9 (10,11), 12,13.
Positive scores—variables 2,3,4,10,11.

Chapter 7

Table 16   *Principal component analysis—A*

Variables	Component I	Component II
Verbal communication (child)	0·41	−0·16
Occupational social class (parent)	0·33	−0·29
Imitation of gestures (child)	0·28	0·13
Right/left differences (child)	0·25	0·15
Specific speech delay (child)	0·21	0·28
English Picture Vocabulary Test (EPVT) (child)	0·45	0·11
Auditory visual integration (child)	0·39	−0·21
WISC scatter (child)	0·30	0·34
Hearing (child)	0·22	0·01
ITPA scatter (child)	−0·02	−0·12
Language literacy index (mother)	0·08	−0·52
Good speech and articulation (of child)	0·09	−0·46
Sex (male) (child)	0·13	0·33
Variance	21%	13%

Table 17   *Principal component analysis—B*

Variables	Component I	Component II
1 Social class	0·11	−0·21
2 Language literacy of mother	0·03	−0·22
3 ITPA representation	0·28	−0·03
4 ITPA automatic	0·28	−0·05
5 WISC performance IQ	0·26	0·19
6 WISC verbal IQ	0·24	−0·05
7 EPVT	0·24	0·09
8 Frostig—visual perception	0·22	0·14
9 Skemp visual concepts	0·23	0·24
10 Harris Draw-a-Man Test (conceptual maturity)	0·20	0·20
11 Imitation of gestures	0·15	0·08
12 Verbal communication code	0·22	−0·22
13 Sentence complexity	−0·22	−0·24
14 Sum of spoken words	0·24	0·28
15 Mean sentence length	0·25	−0·25
16 Renfrew Bus Story content score	−0·26	−0·05
17 Little evidence of use of incomplete sentences	0·09	−0·35
18 Good speech articulation of child	0·07	−0·27
19 WISC scatter	0·12	0·28

(*cont.*)

Table 17 (*cont.*)

Variables	Component I	Component II
20 Cross commands (right/left differentation)	0·13	0·23
21 Simple commands (right/left differentiation)	0·10	0·28
22 Specific speech delay	0·09	0·29
Variance	37·6%	8·8%

Only variables with a loading of 0·09 or more on the first or second component have been included. Sum of spoken words does not necessarily reflect verbal facility or quality of language.

Part II—The hearing-impaired study

Chapter 8

Table 18 *Family and social data*

Features	A = Normal hearing	B = Partially hearing	C = Profoundly deaf	*Significance*		
				A *vs* B	A *vs* C	B *vs* C
Adverse social risk scale (mean score)	1·19	1·28	0·72	NS	1%	5%
Father—satisfactory breadwinner	70%	89%	90%	1%	NS	NS
Family regularly obtained magazine	39%	75%	75%	1%	1%	NS
Father belongs to library	32%	63%	43%	1%	NS	5%
Mother belongs to library	43%	47%	38%	NS	NS	NS
Child belongs to library	53%	58%	25%	NS	1%	2%
Child regularly reads books	61%	68%	22%	NS	1%	1%
Child reads comics	61%	63%	28%	NS	1%	1%
Mother reads to child	67%	83%	83%	NS	NS	NS
Father reads to child	64%	88%	96%	2%	1%	NS

Table 19 Intra-family factors and deafness

		A = Controls	B = Partially hearing	C = Profoundly deaf	Significance		
Feature					A vs B	A vs C	B vs C
		%	%	%			
No disagreement on child rearing		66	84	94	NS	2%	NS
Joint parental decisions on health		23	53	55	1%	1%	NS
Joint parental decisions on finance		35	74	68	1%	1%	NS
Joint husband and wife leisure outings in previous months	0–1	51	11	12	1%	1%	NS
	2–5	32	53	62			
	6–9	17	36	26			
Leisure outing of wife alone in previous months	0–1	49	11	12	1%	1%	NS
	2–5	36	53	62			
	6–9	15	36	26			
Critical remarks by mother about child	none	18	50	42	2%	2%	NS
	few	42	16	45			
	some	28	16	6			
	many	11	16	6			
Positive remarks by mother about child	many	28	72	84	1%	1%	1%
	some	29	28	10			
	few	30	0	6			
	none	12	0	0			

Table 20 *Parent–child interactions*

Feature	A = Control %	B = Partially hearing %	C = Profoundly deaf %	Significance A vs B	A vs C	B vs C
Mother–child communication: regular and daily	88	63	50	2%	1%	NS
Father–child communication: regular and daily	64	50	27	1%	NS	NS
Confiding in parents: usually	62	42	50	5%[a]	5%[a]	NS[a]
Discipline mainly administered by: mother	35	68	71	5%	1%	NS
father or jointly	65	32	29			
Prohibition score 0–5	45	25	21	5%	5%	NS
6–9	55	75	79	almost		
Mothers perception of importance of speech (as needing to be corrected)	65	78	87	NS	2%	NS
Avoidance of baby talk by mother	60	83	34	NS	2%	1%
Expectations (a) Shopping	50	42	25	NS	1%	NS
(b) Usually tidies toys	54	16	22	1%	1%	NS

[a] Based on a 2 × 3 chi-square test

Table 21 *Rankings of mean scores—ITPA*

	Controls		Specific delay		General delay		Partially hearing		Profoundly deaf	
	m[a]	r[b]	m	r	m	r	m	r	m	r
Visual reception	28·9	1	28·7	2	24·3	4	25·8	3	22·9	5
Visual association	31·1	1	29·7	2	26·5	4	29·2	3	26·0	5
Manual expression	32·8	2	31·6	4	29·2	5	31·8	3	34·5	1
Visual closure	30·1	2	29·2	3	24·1	5	30·7	1	24·7	4
Visual seq. memory	33·8	1	31·8	3	29·1	5	32·1	2	29·3	4
Sum of ranks	7		14		23		12		19	
Rank of Index of handicap (See Table III, p. 160)	1		2		3		4		5	

[a] m = mean [b] r = rank
High rankings e.g. 1 or 2 = high achievements
Low rankings e.g. 4 or 5 = low achievements

Table 22 Rankings of mean scores—WISC and other tests

	Controls		Specific delay		General delay		Partially hearing		Profoundly deaf	
	m^a	r^b	m	r	m	r	m	r	m	r
Picture completion	10·8	2	11·7	1	9·9	4	10·0	3	9·3	5
Picture arrangement	9·4	2	8·3	3	7·5	4	9·6	1	7·1	5
Block design	10·5	1	10	3	8·5	5	10·1	2	9·2	4
Object assembly	10·3	2	9·5	4	9	5	10·8	1	10·1	3
Coding	9·8	2	9·1	4	6·9	5	10·8	1	9·7	3
Sum of ranks	9		15		23		8		20	
Frostig	95·9	1	86·8	2	78·8	5	83·4	3	81·9	4
Draw-a-Man	96·4	1	94·9	2	87·3	5	91·4	3	88	4
WISC performance scale	101·2	2	98·9	3	88·6	5	101·9	1	93·6	4
RQ	93·9	1	82·5	3	76·2	4	87·6	2	74·4	5
Sum of ranks	5		10		19		9		17	
Rank of Index of handicap (See Table III, p. 160)	1		2		3		4		5	

^{a} m = mean ^{b} r = rank

Table 23   *WISC verbal scale subtest scores of control, residual speech retarded and partially hearing children*

Tests			Groups		Significance	
WISC		A = Controls	B = Residual speech retarded	C = Partially hearing	A *vs* C	B *vs* C
Information	m	8·7	6·9	6·2	1%	NS
	s.d.	2·2	2·2	2·4		
Comprehension	m	7·2	6·6	5·1	1%	1%
	s.d.	1·9	1·9	2·8		
Arithmetic	m	10·2	9·1	8·2	1%	NS
	s.d.	2·8	2·3	2·4		
Similarities	m	8·9	7·5	5·4	1%	1%
	s.d.	2·3	2·2	2·7		
Vocabulary	m	9·1	7·5	6·5	1%	NS
	s.d.	1·9	1·7	2·5		
Verbal IQ	m	92·5	84·3	76·7	1%	1%
	s.d.	9·9	9·2	13·8		

Table 24   *ITPA verbal subtest scores of controls, residual speech retarded and partially hearing children*

Tests			Groups		Significance	
ITPA		A = Controls	B = Residual speech retarded	C = Partially hearing	A *vs* C	B *vs* C
Auditory reception	m s.d.	33·1 6·8	29·2 6·1	18·6 6·6	1%	1%
Auditory association	m s.d.	33·8 7·5	27·2 7·5	19·4 9·7	1%	1%
Verbal expression	m s.d.	36·9 3·2	33·9 3·37	30·4 3·3	1%	1%
Grammatic closure	m s.d.	36·8 7·6	28·7 7·7	16·0 14·5	1%	1%
Auditory seq. memory	m s.d.	34·1 5·9	29·9 5·2	28·6 4·8	1%	NS

Table 25 Cognitive style data of hearing-impaired, residual speech retarded and normal control groups. Based on principal component analysis

Measures	A = Controls (n = 100)		B = Residual speech retarded (n = 80)		C = Deaf (n = 54)		Significance	
	m[b]	s.d.	m[b]	s.d.	m[b]	s.d.	C vs A	B vs C
Component I (a) 'Mental ability'	1·129	2·073	−0·701	2·617	−1·044	1·150	[a]	NS
Component II (b) 'Motor ability' vs 'Visual-symbolic' ability	0·281	1·091	0·047	0·938	−0·594	1·048	[a]	[a]

[a] statistically significant at the 0·001 level
[b] mean component score

Appendix 2
Description of test materials

First round assessment (first year)

1 *English Picture Vocabulary Test (i)* (Brimer and Dunn, 1962)
This is a test of vocabulary comprehension designed for children between the ages of five years and eight years, eleven months. The test comprises a series of pictures which are arranged in order of increasing difficulty and the child's task is to identify (usually by pointing) one of a choice of four pictures which has been named by the examiner.

2 *Purdue Pegboard* (Tiffin, 1968)
Although this test has not been standardized for children, its authors assert that it is sufficiently simple and straightforward for use with children. It is designed to measure manual dexterity, a function which, they believe, is largely independent of educational level (Rapin *et al.*, 1967).

3 *Frostig Developmental Test of Visual Perception* (Frostig, 1966)
This is a test designed for the assessment of children's visual perception. Each child is provided with a Frostig booklet and a pencil; his task is to complete five different operationally defined perceptual tasks according to the instruction conveyed by the examiner. In the case of the deaf, instructions are mimed.
    The five operationally defined subtests are as follows:

    (i) *Eye motor co-ordination*–the child has to draw continuous straight, curved or angled lines between boundaries of various width, or from point to point with guide lines.
    (ii) *Figure ground*—This involves shifts in perception of figures against increasingly complex grounds; the child is required to discern figures which intersect with other figures by outlining them with coloured pencils.

(iii) *Constancy of shape*—the child has to recognize certain geometric figures (circles, squares, etc.) presented in a variety of sizes, shadings, textures and positions in space, and to discriminate these from similar geometric figures, by outlining the appropriate figures with coloured pencils.

(iv) *Position in space*—the child has to identify an identical object from a set of five orientated differently.

(v) *Spatial relationships*—this involves simple forms and patterns which the child has to copy from a model alongside the page, by using a choice of dots to guide him.

A perceptual quotient score is derived from the total of the scaled scores of the five subtests.

4 *The Illinois Test of Psycholinguistic Abilities: Revised Edition* (Kirk *et al.*, 1968)

The ITPA comprises 12 subtests, each of which allegedly taps a different aspect of language behaviour (Paraskevopoulos and Kirk, 1969; Hare *et al.*, 1973; Newcomer *et al.*, 1974). It has been found to be a useful diagnostic instrument for children with learning difficulties and language handicaps (Olson, 1961; Bateman, 1965; Gerber and Hertel, 1969; Kirk and Kirk, 1971; Marinosson, 1974).

Although the ITPA has been standardized on an American population it has, like the Wechsler Intelligence Scale for Children, been found to be appropriate for use on an English population (Phillips, 1968; Mittler, 1969; Mittler and Ward, 1970; Marinosson, 1974). Mittler (1968) considers the ITPA to be one of the most promising instruments for the assessment of language that has appeared for some time. Elsewhere he points out that there is wide agreement that the test has considerable value for individual clinical investigation (Mittler and Ward, 1970).

The 12 subtests of the revised edition are, in brief:

(i) *Auditory reception*—ability of a child to understand simple questions requiring a yes/no answer.
   e.g. 'Do cats bark?', 'Do babies cry?'

(ii) *Visual reception*—ability of a child to comprehend and recognize the nature of one picture in relation to four other pictures, one of which is similar to that of the stimulus picture. For example, 'See this' (picture of a shoe) 'find one here.'

(iii) *Auditory vocal association*—ability of a child to relate concepts presented orally. This is a type of analogies test, which requires the child to complete the analogy verbally. For example, 'Bread is to eat, milk is to . . .' 'John is a boy, Mary is a . . .'

(iv) *Visual motor association*—ability of a child to comprehend the relationship between visually presented symbols; a kind of visual analogy. For example, the examiner, pointing to four optional picture items (for instance, a knife, a nail, a needle and a screw) briefly in turn, asks the child 'which one of . . . these goes with this one?' (pointing to a picture of a hammer).

(v) *Verbal expression*—ability of a child to express ideas in words. The child is shown various familiar objects (a ball, a wooden block, an envelope and a button) one at a time, and he is asked to tell 'all about' the object.

(vi) *Manual expression*—ability of a child to express ideas by means of manual gesture and pantomime. For example, pictures of common objects (telephone, camera, etc.) are shown one at a time, whereupon the child is instructed to indicate by appropriate gesture and action his knowledge of each object.

(vii) *Grammatic closure*—ability of a child to deal with various grammatical structures concerning comparatives, prepositions, plurals, superlatives and tenses, in relation to pictures portraying the content of certain verbal expressions. For example, 'Here is a *dog*, there are two . . .' 'This boy is *opening* the gate. Here the gate has been . . .' 'This cat is . . .' (*on the chair*).

(viii) *Visual closure*—ability of a child to seek out and identify an incomplete picture item embedded among various other items. For example, the child is shown the picture of a fish and then is asked to find as many fish as possible, in an underwater scene depicting tropical plants and fish variously scattered around.

(ix) *Auditory sequential memory*—ability of a child to reproduce from short-term memory sequences of digits; this is a forward digit repetition test involving digits ranging from 2 to 8 in length, e.g. '7–9'; '8–2–9–3'.

(x) *Visual sequential memory*—ability of a child to reproduce from short-term memory sequence of nonmeaningful geometric figures presented in visual form.

Supplementary test

(xi) *Auditory closure*—ability of a child to hear and fill in a missing part of a word and then to produce that word in complete form. The incomplete word is spoken by the examiner while the child listens and then tries to reproduce the word complete with its missing part. For example, 'airpla/(airplane)'; 'tele/one (telephone)'.

(xii) *Sound blending*—ability of a child to synthesize the separate parts of a complete word articulated by the examiner. For example, 'c – u – p', following which the child should say 'cup'; 'b – a – b – i – e – s = babies', etc.

Scoring

The scoring of the ITPA makes provision for raw scores, scaled scores, a psycholinguistic age and a psycholinguistic quotient.

Modifications to wording of certain subtest items

In keeping with Phillips (1968) and Mittler and Ward (1970), one of the present authors (T. F. in collaboration with senior colleagues in the Nuffield Department) has made appropriate changes to the few 'Americanisms' scattered among the various subtests, because such 'Americanisms' were considered to be unfamiliar to our population of children. Changes include the following:

On Auditory reception:
Item 16	for hatchet	read hammer
	for chop	read bang
Item 30	for barometer	read thermometer
Item 45	for beverages	read liquids

On Auditory closure:
Item 12	for turtle	read tortoise
Item 13	for pound	read bang
Item 21	for pickle	read sausage
Item 29	for pants	read trousers

On Grammatic closure:
| Item 13 | for cookies | read cakes |

On Auditory closure:
Item 11	for / aseball (baseball)
	read / ootball (football)
Item 16	for auto / o / ile (automobile)
	read mo / or / ar (motorcar)
Item 21	for / an / a / aus (Santa Claus)
	read Fa / er Chris / ma / (Father Christmas)
Item 28	for / andy / ar (candy bar)
	read cho / o / ate / ar (chocolate bar)

5 *Draw-a-Man Test* (Harris, 1963)
This is considered to be a useful additional measure of children's cognitive functioning and more specifically, their conceptual maturity. Each child is provided with a foolscap sheet of paper and pencil and instructed to draw a man. On completion of the drawing, the child is given a second sheet of paper with the instruction to draw a woman. The average score from the two drawings is used as this is considered to be a more reliable estimate of the child's performance than reliance on any one of the drawings alone. Emphasis of assessment is placed on *graphic* considerations such as, for example, dimensional representation, proportion and perspective, body parts, clothing, etc., as opposed to artistic merit.

6 *Test of Intersensory Performance* (adapted from Birch and Belmont, 1964; Kahn and Birch, 1968)

This is a test designed to provide some index of the child's ability to integrate sensation from different sensory modalities as shown by his ability to perform tasks emphasizing visual, auditory and tactile responses. It has not been standardized on a representative sample and is without norms; nevertheless it is useful for comparing groups of children of similar age.

In the present study the measurement of intersensory behaviour is based on three interrelated tasks as follows:

(i) *Auditory-visual integration test* The child has to identify a visual dot-pattern that corresponds to the patterning of a rhythmic auditory stimulus. In other words, the child is required to translate an auditory stimulus to a visual response.

(ii) *Haptic-visual integration test* The child has to identify by feel the shapes of different geometric designs which are made of wood and to indicate his response by pointing to a visual equivalent. In other words, the task involves translation of a tactile stimulus into a visual response.

(iii) *Haptic-visual size discrimination test* The child has to discriminate between different-sized objects of the same shape by feel and then to match them by pointing to a replica which is arranged among others of varying size alongside the subject. In other words, he has to translate a tactile stimulus into a visual response.

7 *Measurement of Expressive Verbal Grammatical and Syntactical Ability of Renfrew's Bus Story* (Renfrew, 1971)

Renfrew's Bus Story constitutes a useful stimulus for eliciting a sample of the child's verbal language ability and also his sentence complexity and use of grammatical syntax. Each child's Bus Story was recorded on a tape recorder and then transcribed verbatim on paper for analysis and scoring. To save space only a brief description of scoring is reported here. Full details are available from T.F.

(A) *Number of incomplete sentences.*

(B) *Sentence complexity*—this involved an analysis of complete sentences according to their structural or grammatical complexity. Four types of sentence were classified as follows:

   (i) *Simple sentences*

     That is a sentence without a phrase, or with a phrase used as adjective or adverb in apposition, for example 'The bus ran quickly'.

     A simple sentence is assigned a score of 1

   (ii) *Simple-plus sentence*

     That is a simple sentence with:

(a) two or more phrases, or

(b) a compound subject or predicate with a phrase or predicate and phrase, for example, 'The bus raced down the hill with the driver of the bus'.

A simple-plus sentence is assigned a score of 2

(iii) *Compound sentence*

That is any sentence containing two independent clauses usually joined by a co-ordinating conjunction, 'and', 'but', etc. For example, 'He fell in the pond with a splash and stuck in the mud'.

A compound sentence is assigned a score of 3

(iv) *Complex and/or elaborate compound sentence*

A complex sentence is one which contains one main clause and one or more dependent clauses with:

(a) Noun clause used as: subject, object, in apposition, as predicate nominative, or as objective complement.

(b) Adjective clause.

(c) Adverbial clauses of: time, place, manner comparison, condition concession, cause, purpose, result.

(d) Infinitives.

An elaborate sentence is one which includes more than two independent clauses, or subordinate clauses or phrases. For example, 'When his driver found where he was, he telephoned for a crane to pull him out and asked it to put it back on the road again.'

Either of these sentences is assigned a score of 4

To derive an overall *sentence complexity* score for each child, the number (frequency) of each type of sentence is multiplied by the score for that sentence and the products of these are added together: for example,

3 simple sentences	$= 3 \times 1 =$	3
2 simple-plus sentences	$= 2 \times 2 =$	4
1 compound sentence	$= 1 \times 3 =$	3
3 complex sentences	$= 3 \times 4 =$	12
		—
		22
		—

e.g. Sentence complexity score = 22

(C) *Mean sentence length*

The use of the 'mean length response' index, based on the mean number of words per sentence, is acknowledged by many (Renfrew, 1971; Miner, 1969; Barlow and Miner, 1969, Milgram *et al.*, 1971) to be a relatively satisfactory language performance measurement technique. According to McCarthy (1954) it represents 'a reliable, easily determined, objective, quantitative and easily understood measure of linguistic maturity'.

For the present study the number of words in the five longest sentences of each child's Bus Story constitutes the mean length response index. This is derived from the number of words in the five longest sentences divided by five. For example, number of words in the five longest sentences = 60/5 = 12. Therefore, mean sentence length = 12.

(D) *Information content of Bus Story*

Each child's Bus Story was scored for its 'factual' information in relation to the original version according to the scoring guidelines of Renfrew. Renfrew provides two groups of 'most common responses'; those which comprise the *main* items and those which comprise the *subsidiary* items. The main items comprise 21 features, each of which scores 2 points (or 1 point for half correct). The subsidiary items comprise 13 features and there is a score of 1 point allowed for each of the items which are remembered in context.

8 *Verbal Communication Code of the Child as Reflected in his Bus Story*

The purpose here is to evaluate the verbal communication code or style of each child. The source of material is Renfrew's Bus Story. Each child's version of the story has been tape-recorded and then transcribed on paper verbatim for analysis and scoring. To save space, details of scoring have been omitted, but they are available from T.F. The rules for evaluating the child's communication code are adapted from Bernstein (1961, 1962). He postulates two main codes of communication—the 'restricted' and the 'elaborated', each of which is distinguished according to use of grammar and syntax, organization of ideas and expression of statements.

Communication code/style is rated along a five-point scale as follows:

highly restricted	restricted	moderate	elaborate	highly elaborated
5	4	3	2	1

(The person who rated each child's Bus Story for his communication code was not connected with the research and was acting independently. As such the rating was a 'blind' exercise thus minimizing effects of bias.)

9 *Children's Behaviour Questionnaire: Child Scale 'B' Form* (Rutter, 1967)

This questionnaire has been standardized on a population of English children of both sexes, aged between seven and 13 years. It is described in detail by the authors (Rutter, 1967, Rutter *et al.*, 1970) and has been used extensively in research. The authors report satisfactory levels of reliability.

Second round assessment (second year)

1 *Skemp Visual Concepts Test* (Skemp, 1967)
This test was devised by Dr Richard Skemp and was intended as the first stage of a test battery which ultimately was aimed at including measurement of various cognitive operations in three separate modalities—visual, auditory and haptic. The test used in this study concerns the visual modality and is designed to assess memory, paired association and concept-formation by tests involving memory cards, paired associates and visual concepts, according to the principle of 'learning-to-learn'.

Although Dr Skemp kindly made available the use of his Visual Concepts Test, unfortunately it has not yet been published. However, some relevant data regarding its construction are provided.

The test has been standardized on a normal sample of young English school children of both sexes, controlled for social class according to father's occupation. This has been done by Dr Skemp in co-operation with other English psychologists for the following age groups and sample sizes of children:

> 120 5-year-olds
> 112 5½-year-olds
> 131 6-year-olds
> 136 6½-year-olds
> 139 7-year-olds
>
> Total 638

Tables of norms are provided for each of the three tests—memory cards, paired associates and visual concepts—and for a total score which is calculated in terms of *raw* scores. However, because the mean age of the children in our study was about 7½ years at the time of doing Skemp's Test, his normative data have not been appropriate. As the children tested were of similar age, and because our study was mainly comparative, the norms are fortunately not necessary.

2 *Schonell Graded Word Reading Test* (Schonell and Schonell, 1960)
This test comprises a representative sample of words of increasing difficulty with the aim of providing an index of a child's reading attainment. The more fundamental aspects of reading, such as word recognition and the look-and-say approach, are assessed.

3 *Lateral Dominance Test* (Harris, 1958)
Each child was tested for hand and eye dominance on the basis of the procedures outlined by Harris.

4 *Right–Left Differentiation* (Harris, 1958; Benton, 1968)

According to Alexander (1965) the complex process of right–left differentiation develops over a number of years and is marked by three stages. The first stage, evident between roughly five and nine years of age, sees the acquisition of the child's ability to discriminate right and left with reference to his own body. The second stage, which occurs between eight and 11 years of age, witnesses the child's ability to differentiate right from left on a person facing himself. The third stage, from about 11 years of age, onwards, represents a gradual expansion of right–left directional sense in relation both to objects and to space.

It is the 'first-stage' of right–left differentiation ability with which the present study is concerned—that is, the child's ability to differentiate between right and left relative to his own body.

Each child is required to differentiate first, right from left in relation to *one side* of his body, and second, in relation to *opposite sides,* as follows:

(i) The child is asked:
     'Show me your *right* hand'
     'Show me your *left* ear'
     'Show me your *right* eye'
(ii) The child is asked:
     'Show me your *right* ear with your *left* hand'
     'Show me your *left* ear with your *right* hand'
     'Show me your *right* eye with your *left* hand'

Scoring for the two sets of instructions is the same. Thus a correct set of responses is rated O. An incorrect or confused set of responses is rated 1.

Note: As the nature of this test is highly loaded on verbal instructions, it was not possible to evaluate the deaf children on right-left discrimination.

5 *Imitation of Gestures* (Berges and Lezine, 1965)

The 'Imitation of Gestures' test devised by Berges and Lezine (1965) is an interesting non-verbal, non-symbolic test; it is described as being concerned with the 'proprioceptive and kinesthetic components (muscle and joint sense) which give us information about our body schema' and which form an important part of the child's sensori-motor organization relative to space.

The material used in the present study is adapted from Berges and Lezine's gestures intended for children aged between six and ten years.

It comprises 20 various hand finger movements and entails the examiner manipulating, with his own hands and fingers, the model gesture to be imitated by the child who is then scored for accuracy of the model.

6 *Wechsler Intelligence Scale for Children* (Wechsler, 1949)
Owing to the fact that the WISC is such a well-known and widely used test in research and clinical fields alike, no attempt is made at describing it in any detail. Suffice it to say that 'the theory underlying the WISC is that intelligence cannot be separated from the rest of the personality, and a deliberate attempt has been made to take into account the other factors which contribute to the total effective intelligence of the individual' (Wechsler, 1949).

The composition of the test facilitates assessment of both verbal IQ and performance IQ separately, and a full scale IQ. To arrive at each of these scores a child is given various subtests subsumed under the verbal scale and performance scale, as follows:

verbal scale:	Information
	Comprehension
	Arithmetic
	Similarities
	Vocabulary
performance scale:	Picture completion
	Picture arrangement
	Block design
	Object assembly
	Coding

The two supplementary tests, namely Digit Span and Mazes were not used in the present study.

From the ten subtests outlined above, verbal, performance and full scale IQs were computed in accordance with the scoring procedures laid down by Wechsler. For the majority of deaf children, only the performance scale could be used, in which case instructions were mimed.

The population mean IQ is 100 with a standard deviation of 15.

7 *Junior Eysenck Personality Inventory* (Eysenck, 1965)
This scale is designed to measure the two major personality variables of neuroticism/stability and extraversion/introversion in children. It is adapted from the well-known adult versions, namely the Maudsley Personality Inventory (Eysenck, 1959) and Eysenck Personality Inventory (Eysenck and Eysenck, 1964) and has been standardized on a large population of British school children.

The JEPI comprises 60 questions—to be answered either Yes or No—for example:

'Do you often need kind friends to cheer you up?'
'Do you sometimes get cross?'
'Do you like going out a lot?'

Of these 60 questions, 24 assess extraversion, 24 assess neuroticism, and 12 constitute the lie scale which is meant to accommodate for conscious attempts at faking. It has been constructed for the age range 7–16 years.

No great claims are made for the validity of the test though it would nevertheless seem to have some potential. Eysenck reports, for example, that its administration to a population of children attending a child guidance clinic revealed that 'the group as a whole was very significantly above the standardization group with respect to neuroticism, and that there was a significant difference with respect to extraversion between children showing extraverted symptoms and those showing introverted symptoms'. Although the test is intended to be self-administered, the method adopted by the examiner was to read the statements to the child and record his response. This was in order to minimize difficulties associated with poor reading ability and to ensure reliable and efficient completion of the test by the child.

8 *The Edinburgh Articulation Test* (Anthony *et al.*, 1971)
The test of the children's articulation was administered and assessed by Mrs E. Scanlon, Principal Speech Therapist, Fleming Memorial Hospital for Sick Children. Briefly, in this test the child has to name various picture-objects; his ability to do this is scored on the basis of his consonant and consonant clusters used as appropriate to describe the various objects. Although this test has been standardized on younger children with norms directed at the age levels 3–5·75 years, it is nevertheless a suitable instrument for older children. As the children in the present study were matched for age, and because this is a comparative study, the fact that reliance has had to be put on raw scores rather than on the age-corrected scores of the norms does not affect our study.

Each child was scored for:

(i) Total number of correct responses which can range from 0 to 63.
(ii) Number of immature errors: this is analysed using a modification of Anthony's (1971) qualitative assessment system. Each immature response is given a score of 1, so that the higher the score the greater the number of immature errors.

9 *Educational Achievement Questionnaire*
This is a crude questionnaire devised by one of the editors (T.F.). Its aim was to obtain simple information concerning the child's educational attainment on the basis of the teacher's report. The teachers were not aware of whether the child was a control or study subject and therefore the effects of bias were minimized.

References

Ainsworth, M. and Bell, S. M. (1974). Mother-infant interaction and the development of competence. In *The Growth of Competence* (Connolly, K. J. and Bruner, J. S., Eds.). Academic Press, London and New York.

Alexander, D. (1965). In *A Standardized Road-Map Test of Direction Sense* (Money, J., Alexander, D. and Walker, H. T., Eds.). John Hopkins Press, Baltimore.

Anderson, U. M. (1967). The incidence and significance of high-frequency deafness in children. *American Journal of Diseases in Childhood* **113**, 560–565.

Andrews, G. and Harris, H. (1964). *The Syndrome of Stuttering*. Clinics in Developmental Medicine No. 17. Heinemann Medical Books, London.

Anthony, N., Bogle, D., Ingram, T. T. S. and Isaac, M. W. (1971). *The Edinburgh Articulation Test*. Churchill-Livingstone, Edinburgh.

Atkins, M., Kolvin, I., Neligan, G. A. and Clarke, P. (1976). Neurological assessment. In *Born Too Soon or Too Small* (Neligan, G. A., Kolvin, I., Scott, D. McI. and Garside, R. F., Eds.). Clinics in Developmental Medicine No. 61. Heinemann Medical Books, London.

Barlow, M. C. and Miner, L. E. (1969). Temporal reliability of length-complexity index. *Journal of Communication Disorders* **2**, 241–251.

Bartak, L., Rutter, M. and Cox, A. (1975). A comparative study of infantile autism and specific developmental language disorders: I the children. *British Journal of Psychiatry* **126**, 127–145.

Barton, M. E., Court, S. D. and Walker, W. (1962). Causes of deafness in school-children in Northumberland and Durham. *British Medical Journal* **1**, 351–355.

Bateman, B. (1965). Learning disabilities—yesterday, today and tomorrow. *Exceptional Children* **31**, 167–177.

Beckey, R. E. (1942). A study of certain factors related to retardation of speech. *Journal of Speech Disorders* **7**, 223–249.

Beckwith, L. (1971). Relationships between attributes of mothers and their infants' IQ scores. *Child Development* **42**, 1083–1097.

Bellugi, U. and Klima, E. S. (1972). The roots of language in the sign talk of the deaf. *Psychology Today* June, 61–76.

Belmont, L. and Birch, H. G. (1965). Lateral dominance, lateral awareness, and reading disability. *Child Development* **36**, 57–71.

Benton, A. L. (1964). Developmental aphasia and brain damage. *Cortex* **1**, 40–52.

Benton, A. L. (1968). Right–left discrimination. *Paediatric Clinics of North America* **15**, 747–758.

Berges, J. and Lezine, I. (1965). *The Imitation of Gestures*. Clinics in Developmental Medicine. No. 18. Heinemann Medical Books Ltd., London.

Bernstein, B. (1958). Some sociological determinants of perception: an inquiry into sub-cultural differences. *British Journal of Sociology* **9**.

Bernstein, B. (1961). Social class and linguistic development: a theory of social learning. In *Education, Economy and Society* (Halsey, A. H., Floud, J. and Anderson, C. A., Eds.). Glencoe Free Press, California.

Bernstein, B. (1962). Social class, linguistic codes and grammatical elements. *Language and Speech* **5**, 221–240.

Birch, H. G. and Belmont, L. (1964). Auditory-visual integration in normal and retarded readers. *American Journal of Orthopsychiatry* **34**, 852–861.

Blair, F. X. (1957). A study of the visual memory of deaf and hearing children. *American Annals of Deaf* **102**, 254–263.

Blank, M. (1965). Use of the deaf in language studies: a reply to Furth. *Psychological Bulletin* **63**, 442–444.

Blank, M., Weider, S. and Bridger, W. H. (1968). Verbal deficiencies in abstract thinking in early reading retardation. *American Journal of Orthopsychiatry* **38**, 823.

Bowyer, L. R. and Gillies, J. (1972). The social and emotional adjustment of deaf and partially hearing children. *British Journal of Educational Psychology.* **42**, 305–308.

Bowyer, L. R., Marshall, A. and Wedell, K. (1963). The relative personality adjustment of severely deaf and partially deaf children. *British Journal of Educational Psychology* **33**, 85–87.

Brain, Lord (1965). *Speech Disorders—Aphasia and Agnosia*, 2nd Edn. Butterworth, London.

Brandis, B. and Henderson, D. (1970). *Social Class, Language and Communication*. Routledge and Kegan Paul, London.

Brennan, M. (1976). Can deaf children acquire language? *Supplement to the British Deaf News* February 1976.

Brimer, M. A. and Dunn, L. M. (1962). *English Picture Vocabulary Test*. Educational Evaluation Enterprises, Bristol.

Brodbeck, A. J. and Irwin, O. C. (1946). The speech behaviour of infants without families. *Child Development* **17**, 145.

Brogden, W. J. (1947). Sensory preconditioning. *Journal of Experimental Psychology* **37**, 527–539.

Bronfenbrenner, U. (1976). Is early intervention effective? Facts and principles of early intervention: a summary. In *Early Experience: Myth and Evidence* (Clarke, A. M. and Clarke, A. D. B., Eds.). Open Books, London.

Brown, R. W. and Bellugi, U. (1964). Three processes in the child's acquisition of syntax. In *New Directions in the Study of Language* (Lenneberg, E. H., Ed.). MIT Press, Cambridge, Mass.

Brown, R. and Hanlon, C. (1970). Deviational complexity and order of acquisition in child speech. In *Cognition and the Development of Language* (Hayes, J. R., Ed.). John Wiley, New York.

Brown, R., Cazden, C. and Bellugi-Klima, U. (1969). The child's grammar from I to III. In *Minnesota Symposia on Child Psychology* (Hill, J. P., Ed.) Vol. 3. University of Minnesota Press, Minnesota.

Browne, E., Wilson, V. and Laybourne, P. C. (1963). Diagnosis and treatment of elective mutism in children. *Journal of American Academy of Child Psychiatry* **2**, 605–617.

Bruner, J. S. (1964). The course of cognitive growth. *American Psychologist* **19**, 1–19.

Bruner, J. S. , Oliver, R. R. and Greenfield, P. M. (1966). *Studies in Cognitive*

Growth. Wiley, New York.

Butler, N., Peckham, C. and Sheridan, M. (1973). Speech defects in children aged 7 years: A national study. *British Medical Journal* **1**, 253–257.

Carrier, E. O. (1961). The influence of language in the colour-weight association of hearing and deaf children. *Science and Educational Research Report.* Harvard Graduate School of Education.

Cattell, R. B. (1965). Role of factor analysis in research. *Biometrics* **21**, 405–435.

Cazden, C. (1966). Subcultural differences in child language. *Merrill-Palmer Quarterly* **12**.

Chess, S. and Rosenberg, M. (1974). Clinical differentiation among children with initial language complaints. *Journal of Autism and Childhood Schizophrenia* **4**, 99–109.

Chomsky, N. (1957). *Syntactic Structures.* Mouton, The Hague.

Chomsky, N. (1965). *Aspects of the Theory of Syntax.* MIT Press, Cambridge, Mass.

Chomsky, N. (1969). *The Acquisition of Syntax in Children from 5 to 10.* MIT Press, Cambridge, Mass.

Chovan, W. L. (1972). Role of vocal labelling in memory for object arrangements by deaf and hearing children. *Perceptual and Motor Skills* **34**, 59–62.

Church, J. (1961). *Language and the Discovery of Reality.* Random House, New York.

Clarke, A. D. B. (1968). Learning and human development. *British Journal of Psychiatry,* **114**, 1061–1077.

Cohen, J. (1959). The factorial structure of the W.I.S.C. at ages 7–6, 10–6 and 13–6. *Journal of Consulting Psychology* **23**, 285–299.

Conrad, R. (1976). Matters arising. In *Methods of Communication Currently Used in the Education of the Deaf.* Seminar held from 11th–14th April 1975. Royal National Institute for the Deaf, London.

Conrad, R. (1973). Some correlates of speech coding in the short-term memory of the deaf. *Journal of Speech and Hearing Research* **16**, 375–384.

Conrad, R. (1977). The reading ability of deaf school-leavers. *British Journal of Educational Psychology* **47**, 138–148.

Corah, N. L. and Powell, B. J. (1963). A factor analytic study of the Frostig Developmental Test of Visual Perception. *Perceptual and Motor Skills* **16**, 59–63.

Creak, E. M. (1961). Schizophrenic syndrome in childhood: progress report of a working party (April, 1961). *Cerebral Palsy Bulletin* **3**, 501–504.

Dale, P. S. (1972). *Language Development: Structure and Function.* The Dryden Press.

D'Arcy, P. (1973). *Reading for Meaning. Vol. 1. Learning to Read.* Hutchinson Educational, London.

de Ajuriaguerra, J. (1966). Speech disorders in childhood. In *Brain Function Vol. III: Speech, Language and Communication* (Carterrete, E. C., Ed.). University of California Press, California.

Deutsch, M. (1965). The role of social class in language development and cognition. *American Journal of Orthopsychiatry* **35**, 78–88.

Difransesca, S. (1972). *Academic Achievement Test Results of a National Testing Programme for Hearing-Impaired Students. United States: Spring 1971* (Report No. 9 Series D). Gallaudet College, Office of Demographic Studies, Washington D.C.

Doehring, D. G. and Rosenstein, J. (1960). Visual word recognition by deaf and hearing children. *Journal of Speech and Hearing Research* **3**, 320–326.

Douglas, J. W. B. (1964). *The Home and the School.* MacGibbon and Kee, London.

Douglas, J. W. B., Ross, J. M. and Cooper, J. E. (1967). The relationship between handedness, attainment and adjustment in a national sample of schoolchildren. *Educational Research* **9**, 223–232.

Douglas, J. W. B., Ross, J. M. and Simpson, H. R. (1968). *All our Future: A Study of Secondary Education*. Peter Davies, London.

Eisenson, J. (1966). Developmental patterns of non-verbal children and some therapeutic implications. *Journal of Neurological Science* **3**, 313–320.

Eisenson, J. (1968). Developmental aphasia (dyslogia). A posulation of a unitary concept of the disorder. *Cortex* **4**, 184–200.

Eisenson, J. (1971). Speech defects: Nature, causes and psychological concomitants. In *Psychology of Exceptional Children and Youth* (Cruickshank, W. M., Ed.). Prentice-Hall, New Jersey.

Eysenck, H. J. (1959). *The Manual of the Maudsley Personality Inventory*. University of London Press, London.

Eysenck, H. and Eysenck, S. B. G. (1964). *The Manual of the Eysenck Personality Inventory*. University of London Press, London.

Eysenck, S. B. G. (1965). *Junior Eysenck Personality Inventory (Manual)*. University of London Press, London.

Farber, B. (1960). Family organization and crisis: maintenance of integration in families with a severely mentally retarded child. *Monograph of the Society for Research in Child Development* **25**, 1, Serial No. 75. Antioch Press, Ohio.

Fiedler, M. F., Lenneberg, E. H., Rolfe, U. T. and Drorbaugh, J. E. (1971). A speech screening procedure with three-year-old children. *Pediatrics* **48**, 268–276.

Fisher, B. (1965). The social and emotional adjustment of children with impaired hearing attending ordinary classes. Unpublished M.Ed. thesis, University of Manchester.

Flavell, J. H. (1963). *The Developmental Psychology of Jean Piaget*. Van Nostrand, London.

Fraser, C., Bellugi, U. and Brown, R. W. (163). Control of grammar in imitation, comprehension and production. *Journal of Verbal Learning and Verbal Behaviour* **2**, 121–135.

Freeman, R. D., Malkin, S. F. and Hastings, J. O. (1975). Psychosocial problems of deaf children and their families: A comparative study. *American Annals of the Deaf* **120**, 391–405.

Friedlander, B. Z. (1970). Receptive language development in infancy: issues and problems. *Merrill-Palmer Quarterly* **16**, 7–51.

Friedlander, B. Z. (1971) Listening, language and the auditory environment: automated evaluation and intervention. In *The Exceptional Infant: II Studies in Abnormalities* (Hellmuth, J., Ed.). Bruner/Mazel.

Frostig, M. (1966). *Marianne Frostig Development Test of Visual Perception*. Consulting Psychologists Press, Palo Alto, California.

Fry, D. B. (1966). The development of the phonological system in the normal and deaf child. In *The Genesis of Language: A Psycholinguistic Approach* (Smith, F. and Miller, G. A., Eds.). MIT Press, Cambridge, Mass.

Fundudis, T. (1976) A Psychological Follow-up of Speech Retarded Children. Ph.D Thesis (Unpublished). University of Newcastle upon Tyne.

Furth, H. G. (1961). Visual paired associates task with deaf and hearing children *Journal of Speech and Hearing Research* **41**, 172–177.

Furth, H. G. (1964). Research with the deaf: Implications for language and cognition. *Psychological Bulletin* **62**, 145–164.

Furth, H. G. (1966a). *Thinking Without Language*. Collier Macmillan Ltd., London.

Furth, H. G. (1966b). A comparison of reading test norms of deaf and hearing children. *American Annals of the Deaf* **111,** 461–462.

Furth, H. G. (1971). Linguistic deficiency and thinking: Research with deaf subjects 1964–1969. *Psychological Bulletin* **76,** 58–72.

Furth, H. G. and Youniss, J. (1965). The influence of language and experience on discovery and use of logical symbols. *British Journal of Psychology* **56,** 381–390.

Furth, H. G. and Youniss, J. (1969). Thinking in deaf adolescents: language and formal operations. *Journal of Communication Disorders* **2,** 195–202.

Garside, R. F., Birch, H. G., Scott, D. McI., Chambers, S., Kolvin, I., Tweedle, E. G. and Barber, L. M. (1975). Dimensions of temperament in infant schoolchildren. *Journal of Child Psychology and Psychiatry* **16,** 219.

Gerber, S. E. and Hertel, C. G. (1969). Language deficiency of disadvantaged children. *Journal of Speech and Hearing Research* **12,** 270–280.

Gibson, J. J. and Gibson, E. J. (1955). Perceptual learning: differentiation or enrichment? *Psychological Review* **62,** 32–41.

Glasser, A. J. and Zimmerman, I. L. (1967). *Clinical Interpretation of the Wechsler Intelligence Scale for Children.* Grune and Stratton, New York.

Goetzinger, C. P. and Huber, T. C. (1964). A study of immediate and delayed visual retention with deaf and hearing adolescents. *American Annals of the Deaf* **109,** 297–305.

Goldfarb, W. (1943). Infant rearing and problem behaviour. *American Journal of Orthopsychiatry* **13,** 249–265.

Goodstein, L. D. (1958). Functional speech disorders and personality: a survey of the research. *Journal of Speech Research* **1,** 359.

Graham, P. and Rutter, M. (1970). Selection of children with psychiatric disorder. In *Education, Health and Behaviour* (Rutter, M., Tizard, J. and Whitmore, K., Eds.). Longman Group, London.

Greene, M. (1967). Speechless and backward at three. *British Journal of Disorders of Communication* **2,** 134–145.

Guilford, J. P. (1959). Three faces of intellect. *American Psychologist* **14,** 469–479.

Guilford, J. P. (1967). *The Nature of Intelligence.* McGraw Hill, New York.

Hardy, W. G. (1965). On the language disorders in young children: A reorganization of thinking. *Journal of Speech and Hearing Disorders* **30,** 3–16.

Hare, B., Hammill, D. D. and Bartel, N. R. (1973). Construct validity of selected tests of the I.T.P.A. *Exceptional Children* **40,** 13–20.

Harris, A. J. (1958). *Harris Tests of Lateral Dominance Manual.* The Psychological Corporation, New York.

Harris, D. B. (1963). *Children's Drawings as Measures of Intellectual Maturity.* Harcourt, Brace and World, New York.

Haywood, C. (1967). Experimental factors in intellectual development: the concept of dynamic intelligence. In *The Psychopathology of Mental Development* (Zubin, J. and Jervis, G. A., Eds.). Grune and Stratton, New York.

Hearnshaw, L. S. (1975). Structuralism and intelligence. *International Review of Applied Psychology* **24,** 85–91.

Hebb, D. O., Lambert, W. E. and Lucker, G. R. (1971). Language, thought and experience. *Modern Language Journal* **55.**

Hess, R. D. and Shipman, V. (1965). Early experience and the socialization of cognitive modes in children. *Child Development* **36,** 869–886.

Hewitt, L. E. and Jenkins, E. L. (1946). *Fundamental Patterns of Maladjustment: The Dynamics of their Origin.* Michigan Child Guidance Institute, Springfield, Illinois.

Hine, W. D. (1970). The abilities of partially hearing children. *British Journal of Educational Psychology* **40,** 171–178.

Husen, T. (1975). Social dimensions of the concept of intelligence. *International*

Review of Applied Psychology **24,** 123–130.

Illingworth, R. S. (1966). *The Development of the Infant and Young Child: Normal and Abnormal.* E. & S. Livingstone, Edinburgh and London.

Ingram, T. T. S. (1955). A study of cerebral palsy in the childhood population of Edinburgh. *Archives of Disease in Childhood* **30,** 85.

Ingram, T. T. S. and Reid, J. F. (1956). Developmental aphasia observed in a department of child psychiatry. *Archives of Disease in Childhood* **31,** 161–172.

Ingram, T. T. S. (1959a). Specific developmental disorders of speech in childhood. *Brain* **32,** 450.

Ingram, T. T. S. (1959b). A description of classification of common disorders of speech in childhood. *Archives of Disease in Childhood* **34,** 444.

Ingram, T. T. S. (1963). Delayed development of speech with special reference to dyslexia. *Proceedings of Royal Society of Medicine* **56,** 199.

Ingram, T. T. S. (1969). Developmental Disorders of Speech. In *Handbook of Clinical Neurology* (Vinken, P. J. and Bruin, W., Eds.), Vol. 4. North Holland, Amsterdam.

Ingram, T. T. S. (1972). The classification of speech and language disorders in young children. In *The Child with Delayed Speech* (Rutter, M. and Martin, J. A. M., Eds.). Clinics in Developmental Medicine No. 43, Heinemann Medical Books, London.

Ives, L. A. (1967). Deafness and the development of intelligence. *British Journal of Disorders of Communication* **2,** 96–111.

Jeffree, D. M. (1971). A language teaching programme fo a mongol child. *Forward Trends.*

Jencks, C. (1972). *Inequality.* Basic Books, New York.

Jensema, C. (1975). *The Relationship Between Academic Achievement and the Demographic Characteristics of Hearing-Impaired Children and Youth.* (Report No. 2. Series R) Gallaudet College, Office of Demographic Studies, Washington, D.C.

Jensen, A. R. (1969). How much can we boost I.Q. and scholastic achievement? *Harvard Educational Review* **39,** 1–123.

Jones, H. E. (1954). The environment and mental development. In *Manual of Child Psychology* (Carmichael, L., Ed.), 2nd Edn. John Wiley, New York.

Jones, P. A. and McMillan, W. B. (1973). Speech characteristics as a function of social class and situational factors. *Child Development* **44,** 117–121.

Jordan, T. E. (1962). Research on the handicapped child and the family. *Merrill-Palmer Quarterly* **8,** 243–260.

Kagan, J. and Klein, R. E. (1973). Cross-cultural perspectives on early development. *American Psychologist* **28,** 947–961.

Kagan, J., Rosman, B. L., Day, D., Albert, J. and Phillips, W. (1964). Information processing in the child: significance of analytic and reflective attitudes. *Psychological Monographs* **78** (1, Whole No. 578).

Kahn, D. and Birch, H. G. (1968). Development of auditory-visual integration and reading achievement. *Perceptual and Motor Skills* **27,** 459–468.

Kirk, S. A. and Kirk, W. D. (1971). *Psycholinguistic Learning Disabilities: Diagnosis and Remediation.* University of Illinois Press, Illinois.

Kirk, S. A., McCarthy, J. J. and Kirk, W. D. (1968). *Examiners manual: Illinois Test of Psycholinguistic Abilities* (revised Edn.). University of Illinois Press, Illinois.

Kohen-Raz, R. (1968). Mental and motor development of Kibbutz, institutionalized and home-reared infants in Israel. *Child Development* **39,** 490.

Kolvin, I. and Fundudis, T. (1979). Elective Mutism (In preparation).

Kolvin, I. and Taunch, J. (1973). A dual theory of nocturnal enuresis. In *Bladder Control and Enuresis* (Kolvin, I., MacKeith, R. C. and Meadow, S. R., Eds.).

Clinics in Developmental Medicine, Nos. 48/49. Heinemann Medical Books, London.

Kolvin, I., Ounsted, C., Humphrey, M. and McNay, A. (1971). The Phenomenology of childhood psychoses. *British Journal of Psychiatry* **118**, 385–395.

Kolvin, I., Garside, R. F., Taunch, J., Currah, J., and McNay, R. A. (1973a). Feature clustering and prediction of improvement in nocturnal enuresis. In *Bladder Control and Enuresis* (Kolvin, I., MacKeith, R. C. and Meadow, S. R., Eds.). Clinics in Developmental Medicine Nos. 48/49. Heinemann Medical Books, London.

Kolvin, I., MacKeith, R. C. and Meadow, S. R. (1973b). *Bladder Control and Enuresis*. Clinics in Developmental Medicine Nos. 48/49. Heinemann Medical Books, London.

Kolvin, I., Wolff, S., Barber, L. M., Tweddle, E. G., Garside, R., Scott, D.McI. and Chambers, S. (1975). Dimensions of behaviour in infant school children. *British Journal of Psychiatry* **126**, 114–126.

Kolvin, I., Atkins, M., Barber, L., Tweddle, E. G., Scott, D. McI. and Neligan, G. A. (1976). Behavioural and temperamental assessment. In *Born Too Soon or Too Small* (Neligan, G. A., Kolvin, I., Scott, D.McI. and Garside, R. F., Eds.). Clinics in Developmental Medicine No. 61. Heinemann Medical Books, London.

Kolvin, I., Garside, R. F., Wolstenholme, F., Tweddle, E. G. and Chambers, S. (1978). An abbreviated version of the Maryland Parental Attitude Inventory (for presentation).

Labov, W. (1970). The logic of non-standard English. In *Language and Poverty* (Williams, F., Ed.). Markham, Chicago.

Larr, A. L. (1965). Perceptual and conceptual abilities of residential school deaf children. *Exceptional Children* **23**, 63–66.

Lawton, D. (1968). *Social Class, Language and Education*. Routledge and Kegan Paul, London.

Lenneberg, E. H. (1962). Understanding language without ability to speak: 'a case report'. *Journal of Abnormal and Social Psychology* **65**, 419.

Lenneberg, E. H. (1966). On explaining language. *Science* **164**, 635–643.

Lenneberg, E. H. (1967). *Biological Foundations of Language*. Wiley, New York.

Lenneberg, E. H., Nichols, I. E. and Rosenberger, E. G. (1964). Primitive stages of language development in mongolism. *Procedures of the Association for Research in Nervous and Mental Diseases* **42**, 119.

Leontiev, A. N. and Leontiev, A. A. (1959). The social and the individual in language. *Language and Speech* **2**, 193–204.

Levine, E. S. (1956). *Youth in a Soundless World*. New York University Press, New York.

Levine, E. S. (1960). *The Psychology of Deafness*. Columbia University Press.

Levine, E. S. (1963). Studies in psychological evaluation of the deaf. *Volta Review* **65**, 496–512.

Levine, E. S. (1971). Mental assessment of the deaf child. *Volta Review* **73**, 80–103.

Levine, E. S. and Wagner, E. E. (1974). Personality patterns of deaf persons: An interpretation based on research with the Hand Test. *Perceptual and Motor Skills* **39**, 1167–1236.

Lewis, M. M. (1963). *Language, Thought and Personality in Infancy and Childhood*. Harrap, London.

Lewis, M. M. (1968). Language and Personality in Deaf Children. National Foundation for Educational Research in England and Wales.

Lotter, V. (1966). Epidemiology of autistic conditions in young children: I—Prevalence. *Social Psychiatry* **1**, 124–137.

Lovell, K. and Dixon, E. M. (1967). The growth of the control of grammar in imitation, comprehension and production. *Journal of Child Psychology and Psychiatry* **8**, 31–39.

Luria, A. R. (1961). *The Role of Speech in the Regulation of Normal and Abnormal Behaviour*. Pergamon, Oxford.

MacKeith, R. (1973). Indications for research. In *Bladder Control and Enuresis*. Clinics in Developmental Medicine Nos. 48/49. Heinemann Medical Books, London.

MacKeith, R. C. and Rutter, M. (1972). A note on the prevalence of language disorders in young children. In *The Child with Delayed Speech* (Rutter, M. and Martin, J. A. M., Eds.). Clinics in Developmental Medicine No. 43. Heinemann Medical Books, London.

Marge, M. (1972). The general proglem of language disabilities in children. In *Principles of Childhood Language Disabilities* (Irwin, J. V. and Marge, M., Eds.). Prentice-Hall, Englewood Cliffs, New Jersey.

Marinosson, G. L. (1974). Performance profiles of matched normal, educationally subnormal and severly subnormal children on the revised I.T.P.A. *Journal of Child Psychology and Psychiatry* **15**, 139–148.

Maslow, P., Frostig, M., Lefever, D. W. and Whittlesey, J. R. B. (1964). The Marianne Frostig Developmental Test of Visual Perception, 1963 Standardization. *Perceptual and Motor Skills* **19**, 463–499.

Mason, A. W. (1967). Specific (developmental) dyslexia. *Developmental Medicine and Child Neurology* **9**, 183–190.

Maxwell, A. E. (1959). A factor analysis of the Wechsler Intelligence Scale for Children. *British Journal of Educational Psychology* **38**, 27–37.

McCarthy, D. (1930). The language development of the preschool child. *Institute for Child Welfare Monograph* No. 4. University of Minneapolis Press, Minnesota.

McCarthy, D. (1954). Language development in children. In *Manual of Child Psychology* (Carmichael, 1., Ed.). Wiley, London and New York.

McCarthy, R. J. and Marshall, H. (1969). Memory of deaf and hearing children. *Journal of Genetic Psychology* **114**, 19–24.

McCready, E. B. (1962). Defects in the zone of language (word deafness and word blindness) and their influence in education and behaviour. *American Journal of Psychiatry* **6**, 267–278.

McNeill, D. (1968). On theories of language acquisition. In *Verbal Behaviour and General Behaviour Theory*, (Dixon, T. R. and Horton, D. L., Eds.). Prentice-Hall, Englewood Cliffs, New Jersey.

McQuitty, L. (1957). Elementary linkage analysis for isolating orthological and oblique types and typal relevances. *Educational and Psychological Measurement* **21**, 667–696.

McReynolds, L. V. (1966). Operant conditioning for investigating speech sound discrimination in aphasic children. *Journal of Speech and Hearing Research* **9**, 519–529.

Meadow, K. P. (1968). Early manual communication in relation to the deaf child's intellectual, social and communicative functioning. *American Annals of Deaf* **113**, 29–41.

Meadow, K. P. (1975). The development of deaf children. In *Review of Child Development Research* (Hetherington, E. M., Hagen, J. W., Kron, R. and Stein, A. H., Eds.), Vol. 5. University of Chicago Press, Chicago.

Meadow, K. P. and Schlesinger, H. S. (1971). The prevalence of behavioural

problems in a population of deaf schoolchildren. *American Annals of the Deaf*
116, 346–348.

Menyuk, P. (1964). Comparison of grammar of children with functionally
deviant and normal speech. *Journal of Speech and Hearing Research* **7,** 109–121.

Menyuk, P. (1969). *Sentences Children Use.* MIT Press, Cambridge, Mass.

Menyuk, P. and Looney, P. A. (1972). A problem of language disorder: length
versus structure. *Journal of Speech and Hearing Research* **15,** 264–279.

Meyerson, L. (1963). A psychology of impaired hearing. In *Psychology of
Exceptional Children and Youth* (Cruickshank, W. M., Ed.), 2nd Edn. Prentice
Hall, Englewood Cliffs, New Jersey.

Milgram, N. A., Shore, M. F. and Malasky, C. (1971). Linguistic and thematic
variables in recall of a story by disadvantaged children. *Child Development* **42,**
637–640.

Minde, R. and Minde, K. (1977). Behavioural screening of pre-school children: A
new approach to mental health. In *Epidemiological Approaches in Child
Psychiatry* (Graham, P. J., Ed.). Academic Press, London and New York.

Miner, L. E. (1969). Scoring procedures for the length-complexity index: A
preliminary report. *Journal of Communication Disorders* **2,** 224–240.

Mittler, P. (1968). Psychological assessment. In *Aspects of Autism: Some
Approaches to Childhood Psychoses* (Mittler, P., Ed.). British Psychological
Society, Proceedings of Symposium.

Mittler, P. (1969). Genetic aspects of psycholinguistic abilities. *Journal of Child
Psychology and Psychiatry* **10,** 165–176.

Mittler, P. (1970). Language disorders. In *The Psychological Assessment of Mental and
Physical Handicaps* (Mittler, P., Ed.). Methuen, London.

Mittler, P. (1972). Language development and mental handicaps. In *The Child
with Delayed Speech* (Rutter, M. and Martin, J. A. M., Eds.). Clinics in
Developmental Medicine. No. 43. Heinemann Medical Books, London.

Mittler, P. and Ward, J. (1970). The use of the Illinois Test of Psycholinguistic
Abilities on British four-year-old children: A normative and factorial study.
British Journal of Educational Psychology **40,** 43–54.

Monsees, E. K. (1968). Temporal sequence and expressive language disorders.
Exceptional Children **35,** 141–147.

Moores, D. (1972). Language disabilities of hearing-impaired children. In
Principles of Childhood Language Disabilities (Irwin, J. V. and Marge, M., Eds.).
Prentice-Hall, Englewood Cliffs, New Jersey.

Moores, D. F., Weiss, K. L. and Goodwin, M. W. (1973). Receptive abilities of
deaf children across five modes of communication. *Exceptional Children* **40,**
22–28.

Morehead, D. M. and Ingram, D. (1973). The development of base syntax in
normal and linguistically deviant children. *Journal of Speech and Hearing
Research* **16,** 330–352.

Morley, M. (1965). *The Development and Disorders of Speech in Childhood,* 2nd Edn,
(3rd. Edn. 1972). Churchill Livingstone, Edinburgh.

Murphy, L. J. (1957). *Educational Guidance and the Deaf Child* (Ewing, A. W. G.,
Ed.). Manchester University Press, Manchester.

Myklebust, H. R. (1954). *Auditory Disorders in Children.* Grune and Stratton, New
York.

Myklebust, H. R. (1964). *The Psychology of Deafness,* 2nd Edn. Grune and Stratton,
New York (Reprinted 1971).

Myklebust, H. R. and Brutten, M. A. (1953). A study of the visual perception of
deaf children. *Acta Octolaryngolica Supplementum,* 105.

Neligan, G. and Prudham, D. (1969). Norms for four standard developmental milestones by sex, social class and place in family. *Developmental Medicine and Child Neurology* **11**, 413–422.

Neligan, G., Prudham, D. and Steiner, H. (1974). *The Formative Years: Birth, family and development in Newcastle upon Tyne.* Nuffield Provincial Hospitals Trust, Oxford.

Neligan, G., Kolvin, I., Scott, D.McI. and Garside, R. F. (1976). *Born Too Soon or Too Small.* Clinics in Developmental Medicine No. 61. Heinemann Medical Books, London.

Newman-Keuls Test (1970). In *Statistical Principles in Experimental Design* (Weiner, B. J. Ed.). McGraw-Hill, London.

Newcomer, P., Hare, B., Hamill, D. and McGeffican, J. (1974). Construct validity of the I.T.P.A. *Exeptional Children* **40**, 509–510.

Oleron, P. (1953). Conceptual thinking of the deaf. *American Annals of the Deaf* **98**, 304–310.

Olson, J. L. (1961). Deaf and sensory aphasic children. *Exceptional Children* **27**, 422–424.

Orton, S. T. (1934). Some studies in the language function. *Research Publications of the Association for Research into Nervous and Mental Diseases* **13**, 614–33.

Orton, S. T. (1937). *Reading, Writing and Speech Problems in Children.* Chapman and Hall, London.

Ounsted, C (1955). The hyperkinetic syndrome in childhood. *Lancet* **169**, 303–311.

Ounsted, C. and Taylor, D. C. (1972). *Gender Differences: Their Ontogeny and Significance.* Churchill Livingstone, London.

Paraskevopoulos, J. N. and Kirk, S. A. (1969). *The Development and Psychometric Characteristics of the Revised Illinois Test of Psycholinguistic Abilities.* University of Illinois Press, Illinois.

Pettifor, J. L. (1968). The role of language in the development of abstract thinking: A comparison of hard-of-hearing and normal-hearing children on levels of conceptual thinking. *Canadian Journal of Psychology* **22**, 139–156.

Philip, A. E. and McCullouch, J. W. (1966) Use of social indices in psychiatric epidemiology. *British Journal of Preventive and Social Medicine* **20**, 122.

Phillips, C. J. (1968). The Illinois Test of Psycholinguistic Abilities. *British Journal of Communication Disorders* **3**, 143–149.

Piaget, J. (1952). *The Origins of Intellignce in Children.* International Universities Press, New York.

Piaget, J. (1963). In *The Developmental Psychology of Jean Piaget* (Flavell, J. H., Ed.). Van Nostrand, London.

Piaget, J. (1967). Language and thought from the genetic point of view. In *Psychological Studies* (Elkind, D., Ed.). Random House, New York.

Pless, B. and Graham, P. (1970). Epidemiology of physical disorder In *Education, Health and Behaviour* (Rutter, M., Tizard, J. and Whitmore, K., Eds.). Longman Group, London.

Provence, S. and Lipton, R. C. (1962). *Infants in Institutions.* International Universities Press, New York.

Pumroy, D. K. (1966). M.P.S.R.–Research Instrument with social desirability controlled. *Journal of Psychology* **64**, 73.

Quay, H. D. and Peterson, D. R (1967). *Manual for the Behaviour Problem Checklist.* University of Illinois, Illinois.

Rackstraw, S. J. and Robinson, W. P. (1967). Social and psychological factors related to variability of answering behaviour in five-year-old children. *Language and Speech* **10**, 88–106.

Rainer, J. D., Altshuler, K. Z. and Kallmann, F. J. (Eds.) (1969). *Family and*

Mental Health Problems in a Deaf Population, 2nd Edn. Thomas, Springfield, Illinois.

Randall, D., Reynell, J. and Curwin, M. (1974). A study of language development in a sample of 3 year old children. *British Journal of Disorders of Communication* **9.**

Rapaport, D., Gill, M. M. and Schaffer, R. (1968). *Diagnostic Psychological Testing*, revised Edn. International Universities Press, New York.

Rapin, I., Tourk, L. M. and Costa, L. D. (1967). Evaluation of the Purdue Pegboard as a screening test for brain damage. *Developmental Medicine and Child Neurology* **8,** 45–54.

Reed, M. (1970). Deaf and partially hearing children. In *The Psychological Assessment of Mental and Physical Handicaps* (Mittler, P., Ed.). Methuen, London.

Rees, N. S. (1973). Auditory processing factors in language disorders: The view from Procustes' bed. *Journal of Speech and Hearing Disorders* **38,** 304–315.

Registrar General's Office (1951). *Classification of Occupations*. HMSO.

Reivich, R. S. and Rothrock, I. A. (1972). Behaviour problems of deaf children and adolescents: A factor-analytic study. *Journal of Speech and Hearing Research* **15,** 93–104.

Renfrew, C. E. (1971). *Renfrew Language Attainment Scales*. Churchill Hospital, Oxford.

Rheingold, H. L. (1960). The measurement of maternal care. *Child Development* **31,** 565.

Rheingold, H. S. (1961). The effect of environmental stimulation upon social and exploratory behaviour in the human infant. In *Determinant of Infant Behaviour* (Foss, B. M. Ed.), Vol. I. Methuen, London.

Rheingold, H., Gewirtz, J. L. and Ross, H. W. (1965). Social conditioning of vocalizations in the infant. In *Readings in Child Development and Personality* (Mussen, P. H., Conger, J. J. and Kagen, J., Eds.). Harper and Row, New York.

R.N.I.D. (1976). *Methods of Communication Currently used in the Education of Deaf Children*. Royal National Institute for the Deaf, The Garden City Press, Letchworth, Herts.

Robinson, W. P. (1965). The elaborated code in working class language. *Language and Speech* **8,** 243.

Robinson, W. P. (1969). Social factors in language development in primary school children. In *Proceedings of European Seminar in Sociology of Education* (Mathijssen, M.J.R.M., Ed.). Mouton, The Hague.

Robinson, W. P. and Rackstraw, S. J. (1967). Variations in mothers' answers to children's questions as a function of social class, intelligence test scores and sex. *Sociology* **1,** 259.

Rodda, M. (1970). *The Hearing-Impaired School Leaver*. University of London Press, London.

Rosenstein, J. (1961). Perception, cognition and language in deaf children. *Exceptional Children* **27,** 276–284.

Ross, B. M. (1966). Probability concepts in deaf and hearing children. *Child Development* **37,** 917–928.

Routh, D. K. (1969). Conditioning of social response differentiation in infants. *Developmental Psychology* **1,** 219.

Rutter, M. (1967). A children's behaviour questionnaire for completion by teachers: preliminary findings. *Journal of Child Psychology and Psychiatry* **8,** 1–11.

Rutter, M. (1968). Concepts of autism: A review of research. *Journal of Child*

Psychology and Psychiatry **9,** 1–25.

Rutter, M. (1971). *Infantile Autism—Concepts, Characteristics and Treatment.* Churchill Livingstone, Edinburgh.

Rutter, M. (1972). The effects of language delay on development. In *The Child with Delayed Speech* (Rutter, M. and Martin, J. A. M., Eds.). Clinics in Developmental Medicine No.43. Heinemann Medical Books., London.

Rutter, M. and Graham, P. (1968). The reliability and validity of the psychiatric assessment of the child: I Interview with the child. *British Journal of Psychiatry* **114,** 563–579.

Rutter, M. and Graham, P. (1970). Psychiatric aspects of intellectual and educational retardation. In *Education, Health and Behaviour* (Rutter, M. Tizard, J. and Whitmore, K., Eds.). Longman Group, London.

Rutter, M. and Lockyer, L. (1967). A five to fifteen year follow-up study of infantile psychosis: Description of sample. *British Journal of Psychiatry* **113,** 1169.

Rutter, M. and Martin, J. A. M. (1972). *The Child with Delayed Speech.* Clinics in Developmental Medicine No. 43. Heinemann Medical Books, London.

Rutter, M. and Mittler, P. (1972). Environmental influences on language development. In *The Child with Delayed Speech* (Rutter, M. and Martin, J. A. M., Eds.). Clinics in Developmental Medicine No. 43. Heinemann Medical Books, London.

Rutter, M. and Tizard, J. (1970). Intellectual and educational retardation: Prevalence and cognitive characteristics, In *Education, Health and Behaviour* (Rutter, M., Tizard, J. and Whitmore, K., Eds.). Longman Group, London.

Rutter, M. and Yule, W. (1970). Neurological aspects of intellectual retardation and specific reading retardation, In *Education, Health and Behaviour* (Rutter, M. Tizard, J. and Whitmore, K., Eds.). Longman Group, London.

Rutter, M., Graham, P. and Yule, W. (1970a). *A Neuropsychiatric Study in Childhood.* Clinics in Developmental Medicine, No. 35/36. Heinemann Medical Books, London.

Rutter, M., Tizard, J. and Whitmore, K. (1970b). *Education, Health and Behaviour.* Longman Group, London.

Ruttenberg, B. A. and Wolf, E. G. (1967). Evaluating the communication of the autistic child. *Journal of Speech and Hearing Disorders* **32,** 314–324.

Salfield, D. J. (1950). Observations of elective mutism in children. *Journal of Mental Science* **96,** 1024–1032.

Sattler, J. E. (1974). *Assessment of Children's Intelligence* (Revised reprint). W. B. Saunders, London.

Schein, J. D. (1968). *The Deaf Community: Studies in the Social Psychology of Deafness.* Gallaudet College Press.

Schiff, W. and Dytell, R. S. (1971). Tactile identification of letters: a comparison of deaf and hearing children's performances. *Journal of Experimental Child Psycholoy* **11,** 150–164.

Schlesinger, H. S. and Meadow, K. P. (1972). *Sound and Sign: Childhood Deafness and Mental Health.* University of California Press, Berkeley, California.

Schonell, F. J. (1946). *Backwardness in the Basic Subjects,* 3rd Edn. Oliver and Boyd, Edinburgh.

Schonell, F. J. and Schonell, F. E. (1960). *Diagnostic and Attainment Testing Manual,* 4th Edn. Oliver and Boyd, Edinburgh.

Sheridan, M. (1948). *The Child's Hearing for Speech.* Methuen, London.

Sheridan, M. (1969). Playthings in the development of language. *Health Trends* **1,** 7.

Sheridan, M. (1972). The child's acquisition of codes for personal and interpersonal communication. In *The Child with Delayed Speech* (Rutter, M. and Martin, J. A. M., Eds.). Clinics in Developmental Medicine, No. 43. Heinemann Medical Books, London.

Sheridan, M. (1973). Children of seven years with marked speech defects. *British Journal of Disorders of Communication* **8**, 9–16.

Silverstein, A. B. (1969). An alternative factor analytic solution for Wechsler's Intelligence Scales. *Educational and Psychological Measurement* **29**, 763–767.

Simpson, E. (1964). *The Health of the School Child*, Report of the Chief Medical Officer of the Department of Education and Science, 1962, 1963. HMSO, London.

Skemp, R. R. (1967). Association for Aid to Crippled Children (Visual) Test. Administration manual for tests of visual concepts (Unpublished).

Skinner, B. F. (1957). *Verbal Behaviour*. Appleton–Century–Crofts, New York.

Solomon, A. L. (1961). Personality and behaviour patterns of children with functional defects of articulation. *Child Development* **32**, 731.

Spence, J. C., Walton, W. S., Miller, F. J. W. and Court, S. D. M. (1954). *A Thousand Families in Newcastle-upon-Tyne*. Oxford University Press, Oxford.

Spradlin, J. E. (1968). Environmental factors and the language development of retarded children. In *Development in Applied Psycholinguistic Research* (Rosenberg, S. and Koplin, V. H., Eds.). Macmillan, Riverside, New Jersey.

Stark, J. (1967). A comparison of the performance of aphasic children on three sequencing tests. *Journal of Communication Disorders* **1**, 31–34.

Stott, D. H. (1963). The Social Adjustment of Children (*Manual to the Bristol Social Adjustment Guides*). University of London Press, London.

Streng, A. and Kirk, S. (1938). The social competence of deaf and hard-of-hearing children in a public day school. *American Annals of the Deaf* **83**, 244–253.

Stuckless, E. R. and Birch, J. W. (1966). The influence of early manual communication on the linguistic development of deaf children. *American Annals of the Deaf* **111**, 452–462.

Templin, M. C. (1957). Certain Language Skills in Children. *Institute of Child Welfare Monograph*, No. 26. University of Minnesota Press, Minnesota.

Tiffin, J. (1968). *Purdue Pegboard; Examiner's Manual*. Science Research Associates, Illinois.

Tizard, B. (1971). Environmental effects on language development: a study of residential nurseries. *Paper read at the British Psychological Association Annual Conference, Exeter*, April 1971.

Tizard, J. (1964). *Community Services for the Mentally Handicapped*. Oxford University Press, Oxford.

Tizard, J. (1969). The role of social institutions in the causation, prevention and alleviation of mental retardation. In *Social-Cultural Aspects of Mental Retardation* (Haywood, H. C., Ed.). Appleton–Century–Crofts, New York.

Todd, G. A. and Palmer, B. (1968). Social reinforcement of infant babbling. *Child Development* **39**, 591.

Tramer, M. (1934). Electiver Mutismus bei Kindern. *Z. Kinderpsychiat* **1**, 30.

Treacy, L. (1955). A study of social maturity in relation to factor of intelligence in acoustically handicapped children. Unpublished M.A. Thesis, North Western University.

Trevarthen, C., Hubley, P. and Sheeran, L. (1975). Les activités innées du nourrison. *La Recherche* **6**, 447–458.

US Office of Demographic Studies (1973). *Further Studies in Achievement Testing, Hearing Impaired Students. Data from the annual survey of hearing impaired children and youth* (Series D, No. 13). Gallaudet College, Washington D.C.

Vernon, M. (1961). The brain injured (neurologically-impaired) deaf child: A discussion of the significance of the problem, its symptoms and causes in deaf children. *American Annals of the Deaf* **106,** 239–250.

Vernon, M. (1968). Fifty years of research on the intelligence of the deaf and hard of hearing: A survey of literature and discussion of implications. *Journal of Rehabilitation of Deaf* **1,** 1–11.

Vernon, M. (1969). Sociological and psychological factors associated with hearing loss. *Journal of Speech and Hearing Research* **12,** 541–563.

Vernon, M. (1976). Communication and the education of deaf and hard of hearing children. In *Methods of Communication Currently Used in the Education of Deaf Children.* RNID, England.

Vernon, M. and Koh, S. D. (1970). Effects of early manual communication on achievement of deaf children. *American Annals of Deaf* **115,** 527–536.

Vernon, M. and Koh, S. D. (1971). Effects of oral preschool compared to early manual communication on education and communication in deaf children. *American Annals of Deaf* **116,** 569–574.

Vernon, M. and Miller, W. G. (1973). Language and nonverbal communication in cognitive and affective process. In *Psychoanalyis and Contemporary Science* (Rubinstein, B. M., Ed.), Vol. 2. Macmillan Publishing Co., New York.

Vernon, P. E. (1961). *The Structure of Human Abilities.* Methuen, London.

Vernon, P. E. (1964). *Intelligence and Attainment Tests.* University of London Press, London.

Vernon, P. E. (1969). *Intelligence and Cultural Environment.* Methuen, London.

Wallin, P. (1954). A Guttman scale for measuring women's neighbourliness. *American Journal of Sociology* **59,** 243.

Watson, T. J. (1967). *The Education of Hearing-Handicapped Children.* University of London Press, London.

Wechsler, D. (1949). *Wechsler Intelligence Scale for Children Manual.* The Psychological Corporation, New York.

Weiner, P. S. (1969). The perceptual level functioning of dysphasic children. *Cortex* **5,** 440–457.

Weiner, P. S. (1972). The perceptual level functioning of dysphasic children: A follow up study. *Journal of Speech and Hearing Research* **15,** 423–438.

Werry, J. S. (1972). Psychosomatic disorders (with a note on anesthesia, surgery and hospitalization) In *Psychopathological Disorders of Childhood* (Quay, H. C. and Werry, J. S., Eds.). Wiley, New York.

Whetnall, E. and Fry, D. B. (1964). *The Deaf Child.* William Heinemann Medical Books, London.

Whorf, B. L. (1965). *Language, Thought and Reality.* MIT Press, Cambridge, Mass.

Williams, C. E. (1970). Some psychiatric observations on a group of maladjusted deaf children. *Journal of Child Psychology and Psychiatry* **11,** 1–18.

Wiley, J. (1971). A psychology of auditory impairment. In *Psychology of Exceptional Children and Youth* (Cruickshank, W. M., Ed.). Prentice-Hall, Englewood Cliffs, New Jersey.

Winitz, H. (1966). The development of speech and language in the normal child. In *Speech Pathology* (Rieber, R. W. and Brubaker, R. S., Eds.). North-Holland Publishing, Amsterdam.

Withrow, F. B. (1968). Immediate memory span of deaf and normally hearing children. *Exceptional Children* **35,** 33–41.

Worster-Drought, C. (1965). Disorders of speech in childhood. In *Modern Perspectives in Child Psychiatry I* (Howell, J. G., Ed.). Oliver and Boyd, Edinburgh.

Wrate, R. M., Kolvin, I. and Nicol, A. R. (1978). Reliabilty of a standard psychiatric interview (in preparation).

Wrightstone, J. W., Aronow, M. S. and Moskowitz, S. (1962). Developing reading norms for the deaf child. *American Annals of Deaf* **108,** 311–316.

Yarrow, L. J. (1964). Separation from parents during early childhood. In *Review of Child Development Research* (Hoffman, M. L. and Hoffman, L. W., Eds.), Vol. I. Russell Sage Foundation, New York.

Youniss, J. and Furth, H. G. (1967). The role of language and experience on the use of logical symbols. *British Journal of Psychology* **58,** 435–443.

Yule, W. and Rutter, M. (1970a). Educational aspects of physical disorder. In *Education, Health and Behaviour* (Rutter, M., Tizard, J. and Whitmore, K., Eds.). Longman Group, London.

Yule, W. and Rutter, M. (1970b). Intelligence and educational attainment of children with psychiatric disorder. In *Education, Health and Behaviour* (Rutter, M. Tizard, J. and Whitmore, K., Eds.). Longman Group, London.

Subject index